Because of You

Because of You

Rebekah Gibbs

with Charlotte Ward

headline
review

First published in 2009
by HEADLINE REVIEW

An imprint of Headline Publishing Group

1

Cataloguing in Publication Data is available from the British Library

ISBN 978 0 7553 1888 9

Typeset in Dante by Avon DataSet Ltd,
Bidford-on-Avon, Warwickshire

Printed and bound in Great Britain by
Clays Ltd, St Ives plc

Headline's policy is to use papers that are natural, renewable and recyclable
products and made from wood grown in sustainable forests. The logging and
manufacturing processes are expected to conform to the environmental
regulations of the country of origin.

HEADLINE PUBLISHING GROUP
An Hachette UK Company
338 Euston Road
London NW1 3BH

www.headline.co.uk
www.hachettelivre.co.uk

Photographs from author's collection, except p 3, bottom © BBC;
p 7, top and p 8 © James Vellacott

For Ash and Gigi. My perfect little family.

Contents

Prologue

April 2008

I opened my eyes, blinking sleepily as I tried to focus on the drip in my arm and the drain in my breast. The recovery ward was bright and airy – but that was the last thing I was thinking about as I struggled to work out why I was here.

Then I felt it. A restricted feeling across my chest, not painful, just numb. Now I remembered. I was here because of the cancer. The cancer in my body. The cancer, more specifically, in my breast. The tight feeling constraining me was the bandaging, dressing my wound after a lumpectomy. It meant that the operation was over and the tumour – just under the armpit on my left breast – was gone.

I wanted to feel relieved, but I couldn't. My fight was far from over. Lump or no lump, I still had breast cancer. It was terrifying.

Lying in that hospital bed, which was to be the first of many over the coming months, and trying hard not to cry, I thought back to four weeks ago, when I'd been on a beach in Spain with my fiancé, Ash, and our then seven-week-old baby daughter, Gigi.

I remember thinking at the time how perfect life was, how I'd love to hold on to the moment for ever. I had a great partner and a beautiful daughter. I felt so lucky. As I watched Ash rocking Gigi, I understood the power of a mother's love. This little girl was the centre of my world. She was everything, my reason for being, and I would protect her at all costs.

If only I could have gathered up that feeling and bottled it – because, boy, would I need it in the coming weeks, as my perfect world came crashing down around me.

Little did I know that, at the time my baby needed me most, I'd be diagnosed with an aggressive form of breast cancer and dragged to hell and back as I fought to live.

Who would have thought that, with me aged thirty-five, my carefree world would be thrown into chaos and I'd be forced to stare mortality in the face? That within weeks of becoming a proud new mum, cancer would threaten to rob me of the chance to see my daughter grow up? Well, that's what was happening to me now. Lying in the recovery ward just after the operation, I decided this would be about life, not death.

It was time to get ready for the fight of my life . . .

1. A Poison Within

'If this lump turns out not to be a tumour, I'll buy you a bottle of champagne.'

I almost laughed at the consultant's words. You know when there's a little bit of hope, and you know when the odds are stacked against you. Right then, I knew that, for me, it was the latter.

I was in a private clinic, in Tunbridge Wells. I must have looked a right old state – unkempt, with a shell-shocked expression, holding a crying baby in her car seat, a changing bag and all the other bits and bobs that go with having a newborn. I had just begged the receptionist to give me an appointment to see Mr Williams, a consultant who had been treating my close friend Madeleine for breast cancer.

It was mid-afternoon on a sunny March day, and I'd rushed to the clinic in a panic after a visit to my local doctor that morning. It had been my third visit to my GP's in as many months and, this time, it had resulted in her telling me that she was very concerned about the lump I had noticed in my left breast. It had been there since December, and had been dismissed by my GP and by a locum doctor as nothing but a blocked milk duct – nothing to worry about. I'd tried not to think about it, but I had known something more was wrong: the lump was far too alien not to mean trouble.

'What happens now?' I asked the consultant, biting my bottom lip.

'Well, do you have private healthcare?'

'No,' I answered meekly.

'In that case, I'll see you at the local hospital the day after tomorrow,' he said. 'We'll do a biopsy and an ultrasound scan so that we can find out more. But, I have to say, from the feel and look of it, I will be very surprised if the tumour is not malignant.'

'Right,' I said slowly. I was trying to take it all in. In the space of less than five hours, things had escalated from a simple appointment with my family doctor to a consultant talking about a biopsy.

My thoughts were disturbed by my nine-week-old daughter, Gigi, who was getting a bit grizzly, lifting me out of thoughts about myself. She looked tired and grumpy. We'd dashed here straight from our first doctor's appointment, and she needed feeding and her nappy changing.

I instantly felt guilty. Personal crisis or not, she was uncomfortable, and I had to deal with it before she really started screaming.

I noticed the nurse who'd been in the room while the consultant talked to me – she was looking at me sympathetically. Her concern made me anxious; she must suspect the worst.

'Would you like to go and sit in the consultation room?' she asked me kindly.

'No, I'm fine thanks,' I replied, taking Gigi out of her car seat but desperate to escape.

It was only when I stepped out of the office and headed into the waiting room that I realized I was far from OK. I couldn't breathe properly, and it took all my strength to put one foot in front of the other. I just wanted the whole thing to go away.

I've got cancer. Christ. I've got cancer: I couldn't stop myself saying it, over and over in my head. People with cancer die.

I dashed across the room and headed down the corridor towards the car park. It seemed endless and, by the time I'd reached the exit, I couldn't control my tears. I sped through the sliding doors, passing a father holding his son. Even the knowledge that other people could see me crying didn't change things: I couldn't hold back.

I dialled my fiancé, Ash's, number and told him, still in tears, what the doctor had said. My whole body shook as I spoke to him, trying at the same time to put the car seat, and Gigi, into the car.

Poor Ash. I could barely get the words out, and he was struggling to understand what I was saying in between my sobs.

'Oh, Becks,' he said but, after that, words failed him. He must have felt like he had been punched in the gut and, like me, at that stage, he didn't even begin to know how to make positive noises. He offered to come and pick me up, but it seemed pointless, as I was already in the car and was only a short distance away.

Back home, I didn't know what to do. Gigi was starving, but the last thing I wanted to do was get my breast out and start feeding her. There was something alien and poisonous growing in there, but the milk I was producing was supposed to be the very thing that would keep my baby healthy. I couldn't get my head round it. It felt as if everything had turned upside down.

I fed Gigi reluctantly; she was so hungry there was nothing else I could do.

When Ash stepped through the door, he looked pale with the shock. He walked up to me and hugged me. We stood there without saying a word for what seemed like ages. There didn't seem anything *to* say, a first in all our sixteen years together. In the months that were to follow, we would have a fair few moments like this. It just felt as if our perfect life had been shattered, as if a bomb had gone off right in the middle of it all. This is awful, I thought. It's actually happening to us, to *me*.

After his initial, stunned silence, however, Ash was doing his best to be philosophical.

'We'll just wait until Wednesday, Beck,' he said. 'We

don't know all the facts, but you're young and healthy. You can fight this.' He was looking at me when he said this and, as much as he tried to hide it, I could see the fear dancing in his eyes. 'We'll just have to wait and see exactly what we're up against, and then all we can do is hope for the best.' There are times when clichés can be comforting.

And hoping is what we've been doing ever since cancer crept into our lives. You just wait until the next recovery stage, the next milestone you can tick off the list, the next turning point that brings you one step closer to normality. Except, of course, nothing is ever normal again. That's the bit they don't tell you. Your life changes completely with the diagnosis; and it will never be the same again. But, at this stage, being positive and taking things bit by bit was all we could do. That was the only way to get through it.

Neither of us slept at all that night. I lay in bed, constantly running my fingers over the lump in my breast. It made me feel sick to touch it, but I couldn't stop myself. How could something so small cause me so much worry and stress? Why had it taken Madeleine's diagnosis for me to start making a fuss about this lump? Why had I allowed it to grow and take root? And had I left it too late?

The following day was April Fool's Day; not only that, but every time I looked out of the window, I'd see one bloody magpie in the middle of the garden: one for sorrow.

'I swear it's taunting me,' I huffed to Ash after I'd seen it for the umpteenth time. So he ran outside to scare it off.

After another restless night, and two days after my initial consultation with Mr Williams, I arrived at the local hospital to have my biopsy and ultrasound scan.

It may sound weird, but I had taken a lot of care getting ready; it somehow seemed important that I felt good about myself – despite the potentially devastating news I was facing. I'd even curled my long, brown hair, which has been my pride and joy since my teenage years. As I did so, I wondered if I would lose it soon, wondered if Ash would still fancy me without my trademark hair which he so loved, if Gigi would recognize me without it. Then I quickly filed those thoughts away for another day. One step at a time, Beck.

My friend Charlotte accompanied me for moral support. I'd asked Ash to stay at home to look after Gigi. I'd never left her for longer than half an hour before, so it was reassuring to know that she was safe with her daddy. He'd offered to come, but I insisted I'd be fine. I didn't want him fussing. I felt that keeping the situation low-key would somehow make the outcome a positive one. Just goes to show how you clutch at straws in times of crisis.

At the hospital, I was called in to see Mr Williams, who asked me how I was.

'Have you had any sleep?' he asked.

'Not much,' I admitted.

'Well, I'm not surprised.' He smiled at me. 'It's difficult news to take in. Do you need a moment to get yourself together?'

'No, no, I'm fine. Let's get it over with,' I replied.

I was sent off to the X-ray department, where I was met by Mr Flannigan, who was to perform my biopsy.

Once I'd stripped to the waist – I wondered how many different people I'd be revealing myself to over the next few weeks – I had to lie on the bed, holding my arm up.

Mr Flannigan, assisted by a female nurse, put a cold gel on the area where the lump was, and on my armpit. Then he moved the scanner over my skin and studied what looked to me like a scramble of faint grey shapes on a screen next to him.

I scrutinized his face, trying to read his expression. 'Are you worried?' I asked him. 'Off the record?'

He looked at me with kind eyes. 'I can't say,' he told me apologetically.

I reckon I'm quite good at reading faces, and I was sure there was a slightly sad, sympathetic look in his eye.

The biopsy itself was pretty unpleasant. I didn't know that, once they've found a lump in your boob, they take a biopsy under the arm to test the lymph glands as well, and I instantly started to panic. This was serious.

The needle hurt as it entered the skin of my armpit, and the tears welled.

Afterwards, I was ushered into a room which contained four chairs and a box of tissues, and told to wait to see Mr Williams. I knew he was in the other room talking to Mr Flannigan. It was only five minutes, but the wait was painful.

'I know,' I kept saying to Charlotte, who was trying her hardest to keep me upbeat, 'I know exactly how this is going.'

The whole situation seemed surreal; I felt detached, as if it wasn't me but someone else at the centre of it. I've got a newborn baby, I thought. She's only nine weeks old. How can I have cancer? I kept telling myself that I was young, that young people don't get cancer – they certainly don't *die* of cancer – that I was healthy, I'd be fine. I was thirty-five, for Christ's sake – of course I'd be fine.

But none of this made a scrap of difference. Mr Williams came in and closed the door behind him. He didn't beat around the bush.

'We have a very, very strong suspicion . . .' he said gravely, then he handed me a leaflet entitled 'What do you know about breast cancer?'

I tried to turn the leaflet over in my hands to look at it, but I couldn't even hold it properly, my whole body was shaking so much.

'I think you've got it,' he told me.

I sat there staring at him, unable to get the words out. I was numb with shock but, at the same time, not surprised at all. I actually felt relieved, in a strange way, as if, now that the diagnosis had been made, I was entering into a system that would sort it all out. I felt as if the consultant was saying, 'You're on a list, you're a patient. We're looking after you now. We can make it all go away.'

I wanted to ask, 'So have I got it, definitely?' but, although I said this in my head several times, I couldn't quite bring myself to say it out loud. After I had said it and received an affirmative reply, there would be no going back. I wouldn't be in control.

But there was no escaping the grim reality of the situation. Mr Williams was soon telling me everything I didn't want to hear but needed to know.

'We can't be a hundred per cent sure – we have to wait for the biopsy – but, in our opinion, you have breast cancer,' he said. 'The biopsy results will come through in a week's time and, if they confirm our suspicions, then you'll need an operation to remove the lump.'

We were then joined in the consultation room by Sue, a nurse who specialized in the treatment of patients suffering from cancer, who handed me a prescription for bromcriptine.

'It's to dry your milk up before the operation,' she explained matter-of-factly.

I just thought, Woah! Slow down. I was trying to think positively, and now I was set to embark on a conversation I really didn't want to have. I was a new mother, my job was to feed and nurture my baby, to protect her, and now I wasn't even going to be allowed to do that. I felt light-headed.

Mr Williams went on. 'I think we've found it at the early stages,' he said. 'But if the cancer cells have spread, we might need to do a bigger operation, to remove the breast itself . . .'

Now I was feeling dizzy. The thought that I may have to have a mastectomy left me barely able to focus on what the consultant said next. '. . . lumpectomy, chemotherapy, radiotherapy . . .' None of his words was making any impact.

Thankfully, Charlotte, next to me, was painstakingly making notes, which she later relayed to Ash. I will always be grateful to her for how amazingly strong she was that day – it must have been dreadful for her to experience all that fear and upset first-hand. Now, my appointment over, my only thought was to get back home to Gigi as quickly as possible. All I wanted to do was to hold her tightly and feel her little warm face pressed against my cheek, to shut out the rest of the world. Instead, we had to sit and wait outside the hospital chemist's for my bromcriptine for a torturous thirty minutes.

While I was waiting, I rang Ash to fill him in on what had happened. 'They think it is cancer; in fact, they're almost definitely sure it is,' I said.

'What do you mean, they're almost sure?' he asked.

'Babe, you know what I'm saying – please try and get your head round it,' I said softly. 'It's breast cancer. That's it.'

Next, I called Mum and Dad. Poor Mum just couldn't take it in. I kept the conversation as factual as I could and told her I would call back later that night when I got home. I put the phone down, knowing I had left her upset and worried sick, but I had to get my own head round the situation, and one way of doing this was to let everyone know. And it would be one chore over with. I called my closest friends then and there; I just wanted to hear their voices. I've never needed my friends and family so much in my life.

One by one, they all broke down on the phone when I told them, and I found that I was the one who was being upbeat. 'It'll be all right,' I told them. 'Please don't worry about it. It has just got to be fine.'

On my way home from the hospital, I started to think about the cancer storyline I'd been involved in when I'd played the part of Nina, a paramedic, on the BBC TV show *Casualty*. In it, my onscreen sister was diagnosed with cancer, and my character was her main source of support. That storyline had made me realize that the people around the person with cancer are affected almost as much by it as the sufferer herself. Ash, my parents, my brother, my friends – this is what they would all have to go through now.

Bizarrely enough, my role as Nina had been pretty much my first experience of a hospital environment. In character, all the medical speak would trip off my tongue, but I'd never even so much as been in hospital to have my tonsils out. I'd never really understood what an impact being involved with hospitals and doctors actually had on people and their lives; I'd been able to leave the chaos behind at the end of the day. But I couldn't leave this behind. This wasn't about saying lines that had been put into my mouth by a scriptwriter. The cameras weren't rolling. This was real.

Back home, I tried to cheer myself up with a glass of champagne – weird, given that there wasn't anything to celebrate – but, inside, I felt as if my whole body was aching.

I love my new baby and I love Ash, I thought. I don't want this to be happening. I didn't think, Why me?, at that stage, I was just too blown away by the shock of it all.

Over the next few days, I tried to make myself feel positive, but it was hard work. You're on tenterhooks the whole time. Ash was putting a brave face on things, too, but I could tell he was worried sick, like me.

There were lots of loaded silences, lots of tiptoeing around each other and lots of Ash telling me it would all be fine. He was being so positive that I had to try and talk myself into being positive too. I felt I owed it to him. For Ash, I wonder if having to be upbeat for me meant he somehow talked himself round too, if lifting me up helped to convince him we would get the happy ending we so desperately wanted and needed.

And, of course, none of the everyday stuff stopped. I'd had to have a crash course in feeding Gigi formula from a bottle and, although she'd taken to it fine, she was clearly finding it harder to digest. She hadn't had a poo in days, so she wasn't too happy, and I was concerned.

It would be six days from the date of my last appointment with the consultant before I got the results which would officially reveal what lay in store for me. The weather was lovely, but I felt low, unable to appreciate anything. To me, spring had always signalled the beginning of a new chapter – but this was definitely not what I'd had in mind.

I tried to put the consultant's words to one side and take strength from stories I had heard of people who'd had biopsies and been fine. After all, it wasn't definite that I actually had cancer – it could still be that blocked milk duct.

Cards and flowers were arriving from well-meaning friends, with long, sympathetic messages, but nobody, actually, really knew what to say. My milk was drying up, and the bromcriptine made me feel terrible, really heady and weak.

With that, and the shock, I felt a bit delirious, but there was no time to sit and feel sorry for myself. I still had a baby, and she consumed me. There simply wasn't time to wallow about in self-pity, contemplating my own mortality. Every day, Gigi was doing something new, and it was almost as if she knew something was up: she was sleeping through every night and amusing herself more during the day, rather than needing to be picked up all the time.

When the weekend arrived, I did feel a little better. The Saturday before my results were due was the day of the Grand National, at Aintree. Ash and I always had a little bit of a flutter and, now, more than ever, I felt like trying my luck and placing a bet.

When Ash and I were studying the names of the horses running in the paper, one jumped out at us: Comply or Die.

'Well, that's my situation all over!' I grimaced.

Ash went straight off to the bookies and, after lunch, we settled down in the front room to watch the race on television.

'What colour is my one, babe?' I asked.

'That's it there, Beck!' Ash shouted excitedly, pointing at the screen. 'The one at the front!'

Both of us whooped and cheered as Comply or Die romped to victory. It was nice to be laughing again, and I won £180 to boot! As silly as it sounds, that win really made me feel that things were looking up – surely this was a sign that luck was on my side?

And, in a double victory, Gigi finally had her poo. Thatta girl!

★ ★ ★

Two days later, on 9 April, ten days after my first visit to Mr Williams at the cancer clinic, I was back at the hospital for my results.

Ash and I had tried really hard not to talk about it the evening before, and had tossed and turned in bed that night, but now there was nothing to do but face the situation.

At the clinic, we were met by the same cancer-specialist nurse, Sue, who I had seen the week before and I was ushered into a consulting room. She gave it to me straight.

'You have got cancer,' she told me. 'Grade-three.'

Ash reached out for my hand, but we couldn't look at each other. When he began asking Sue some questions, I could hear the pain in his voice.

'Is there a grade four?'

'No,' she replied.

'Can we survive this?' he added.

'It's possible – some people have,' came the blunt response.

All I knew was that my friend Madeleine was fighting grade two, and that grade-three was very aggressive. I certainly didn't need to look up the statistics on the internet to know that I might not make it.

Then the nurse asked Ash how he was feeling.

He couldn't answer, of course he couldn't; the pain was too much. This was it. I had breast cancer. Our carefree days were over.

There was a long silence, and then I saw that he was

looking at the floor, weeping. He looked like a little boy. For the very first time in the sixteen years we had been together, I saw a vulnerable side to him, and it broke my heart. For once, he didn't know what to do. It took all my strength not to take him in my arms, curl up on the floor with him and cry like a baby too.

Instead, I squeezed Ash's hand tight and listened as Sue went on to explain that I'd need a lumpectomy (an operation to remove the tumour), chemotherapy, radiotherapy and a course of drug treatment, either herceptin or tamoxifen, depending on which I was most compatible with.

She was trying to reassure us, saying that we were now in the system, and explaining what the next procedure would be. Ash asked a few more questions and, when she'd answered them all, we got up to leave, dazed, and made our way home.

The car ride back was mostly silent, but punctuated with Ash trying to be upbeat, giving me a pep talk, telling me that, now we knew what we were dealing with, we could fight it with everything we had. Together.

Those first few days after the biopsy result, we were like two little bunnies with these massive lights shining in our eyes. We were shattered, shocked, petrified and numb, all in equal measures. You know – juggling a baby, with all those hormones popping, and the tiredness, with the bad news, people's sympathy and good wishes. We didn't really know if we were coming or going. But there's only so long you can be beaten and broken. We very quickly realized we would have to find some resolve and launch ourselves into battle. It was time to fight and win the war . . .

2. 'Remember My Name'
– Fame Days

Lying in bed in the dark, I wiped away the tears.

I could hear Gigi breathing, fast asleep in her cot at the end of the bed. Ash, too, next to me, was out for the count, snoring. In some way, I think I hoped that our all being together in the same room would bring me some much-needed comfort. But it didn't – nothing really did.

As I lay there, my eyes stinging, I began to feel really cross with myself. What good would crying do?

What I needed was lots of rest, not to work myself up into a sobbing wreck in the middle of the night.

For me, it's the silence that really does it. There is no more frightening or lonely time than three in morning. It's just you and your thoughts – bleak thoughts about dying and leaving those you love the most. And it wasn't just the thought of dying that scared me – it was the whole unknown business of having cancer. The operation was looming and, the more I found out about it, the worse it sounded. Surgical scars, drains in my breast, rounds of exercises several times every day afterwards to guard against paralysis – and then there was the treatment itself. All that poison I would have to have pumped into my body in order to cure the cancer. I wasn't sure that I could face it, that I was strong enough to get through it all, step by step. It seemed like the biggest uphill struggle, and I felt exhausted before I'd even started.

I became aware that Ash was stirring.

'What's up, Becks?' he asked, in a hoarse voice. Then he sat up sleepily to comfort me. I just shook my head, words failing me, as they did more and more these days.

'Look, babe,' he whispered, pointing to Gigi, fast asleep in her cot. 'Look at her. She's amazing! That's what we've got to live for. That's what you've got to be happy about. You're doing good!'

Snuggling up against him, I sighed and closed my eyes, feeling comforted and determined. What would I do without my Ash? I feel blessed to have him. He just stepped up to this, as he always has with everything else. And I love him even more for it.

When I first met Ash, I was nineteen. He was twenty-six.

Looking back now, it's a wonder either of us pulled that night, as we both looked a little bit ridiculous.

That evening, I'd gone out in a red power trousersuit, complete with ghastly shoulder-pads. Well, it *was* 1993, and that look was all the rage!

I loved that River Island suit. I still have it now and,

every so often, I get it out to see if I can still squeeze into it, then I mince around the house pretending I'm in a Duran Duran video – but that's a whole different story.

Back then, I was living in a tiny little flat in Sidcup and had just finished a stint performing in the *Rocky Horror Picture Show*, where I'd understudied the part of Janet to the actress Liz Carling and was also a phantom in the chorus.

It had been great fun, but now I was between jobs, 'resting', as it's known in the biz, and I couldn't help but fear that being picked for the *Rocky Horror Picture Show* might just have been beginner's luck and that I was a one-hit wonder. I could just about pay my rent with my meagre income from waitressing, and I was spending my time auditioning, partying and trying to mend my broken heart after my last romance, with a very unsuitable boy, had bitten the dust.

That night, I'd met up with Alison Forbes, a good friend from the performing arts college I'd previously attended in Sidcup, who was also 'resting'. We'd agreed to judge a dancing competition in Tunbridge Wells, where Alison lived, in return for a small fee.

For a few months now, we'd been scraping round for every penny (we were both on the dole for a while as well – thankfully, the first and the last time for me) and praying that our theatrical careers weren't over almost as soon as they'd begun.

To be honest, I was feeling a bit lost. It could be pretty

depressing sometimes, especially as all our friends from college were starting to get work around us. Even so, we figured there was no point staying at home, moping. Instead, we'd go out with a fiver in our pockets and drink Diet Coke all night. We were both silly enough to have a laugh without booze anyway.

That night, once we'd done the judging, we'd decided to go on to a cheesy nightclub in Tunbridge Wells called Da Vinci's. And it was there that I first clapped eyes on the delectable Ashley Pitman.

At first, however, he caught my eye for all the wrong reasons.

Nudging Alison, I pointed to where a group of lads was sauntering across the dance floor with all the attitude and confidence of the Jets in *West Side Story*. It was quite a sight. And there, in the middle of this posing pack of testosterone, was an absolute vision in an eye-watering lilac silk jacket.

'Ooh, gorgeous,' murmured Alison, and we both sniggered.

But, underneath that revolting jacket (which I'm sorry to say that, years later, I sneakily chucked away), was a really dashing guy. He was tall, dark and handsome, and very manly – just the way I liked them.

And, as Alison and I stood there giggling at him, he caught my eye and smiled at me coolly (well, as coolly as you could, wearing a silk lilac jacket, I guess!).

I grinned back flirtily, and Alison rolled her eyes and headed off to the bar.

There was a bit of a stand-off to begin with, as neither of us would make the first move. I was standing there, flicking my waist-length hair and mouthing, 'Come over,' but he just smiled back confidently, shaking his head and saying, 'No, you come here.' He obviously wasn't giving in (typical Mr stubborn Gemini) so, after about five minutes of this carry-on, I relented and wandered over to him.

Ah, but you're not getting off that lightly, I thought to myself, giving him a pursed-lipped smile. Now, who can I be?

You see, for fun, I'm always slipping into different characters – usually just to amuse myself. Sometimes, I'll phone British Gas with a brash American accent, all *Guys and Dolls*; other times, I'll be a proper yokel Devon lass – whichever dialect takes my fancy. It used to drive Ash to distraction, but I think he's finally got used to it now, and Gigi adores it, especially if I accompany it with a funny little dance.

But, at the time, Ash knew nothing about me or that I'd playfully decided to wind him up. Gazing down at my red power suit, I had the perfect ruse in mind for this lavender lovely. I decided to be French.

With hindsight, claiming my name was Françoise and that I came from Boulogne – the town featured in my GCSE French textbook – was hardly the most sexy persona I could have come up with. If I'd had more time, perhaps I would have invented Nicole, the gorgeous ballet dancer from Paris, or Darcy, the fashion buyer for Yves Saint-Laurent, but, still, presenting myself as a little French fancy with a sexy purr of *'Bonjour!'* seemed to work a treat.

As I'd hoped, Ash didn't speak a word of my fake native tongue, and you should have seen his eyes light up! I could actually speak very little French myself, but it didn't really matter: Ash had fallen for it hook, line and sinker.

Smiling sweetly, I mixed pidgin French with heavily accented attempts at English.

'Oui! I like the, Laundun . . . 'ow you say? Telefone bax?' I giggled, while Ash gazed at me, completely enthralled.

I was soon straining under the limitations of my very basic conversational French and extremely grateful that Ash appeared to be none the wiser.

'Would you like a drink?' he offered.

'Je voudrais une timbre!' ('I would like a stamp!') I replied enthusiastically.

'Where did you get your suit from, it's very nice!' he continued, speaking loudly and slowly, in the way you might to a deaf person.

'Où est la poubelle?' ('Where is the dustbin?') I smiled sweetly back.

I was able to continue with this charade for a good half an hour – even when Alison headed over to join us. Well aware of my penchant for inventing impromptu characters, she immediately backed me up and pretended that we'd met through a French exchange trip. We painted a picture of an idyllic friendship which had progressed from us being dedicated pen-pals to now meeting up whenever we could.

Ash was clearly loving the little French act. He kept mouthing things to his mates and trying his hardest to impress me.

'You are very pretty,' he said, continuing to speak very loudly and slowly and pointing at my face. I pouted back, shaking my head.

'*Je ne comprends pas, monsieur,*' I exclaimed. 'I do not understand!'

Then, with a big grin on his face, Ash announced, 'I'll come over. And see you. On the boat!' all the time making wave motions with his hand.

He was being so sweet and enthusiastic that I began to feel a bit mean. It had got to the point where I'd had enough of keeping up the act. He seemed like a nice guy, and I wanted to cut to the chase, to tell him, 'I'm actually called Rebekah and I live in Sidcup.' Then we could get on with the night. I thought he'd laugh about it but, when I switched to my normal accent, giggling, he stared at me coldly.

'You're joking,' he said. Then he beckoned to his friends and they strolled off, like a pack of lions, leaving me standing there, feeling very foolish.

Oh God, I've blown it, I thought to myself.

After that, Ash avoided me for the rest of night. I kept

trying to catch his eye, raising my eyebrows at him, but he just gave me the cold shoulder.

I was determined to have a good night, and hit the dance floor with Alison but, secretly, it bothered me. Even though I was having fun, I was constantly aware of where Ash was in the club and hoping that I might get the chance to speak to him again.

Years later, he admitted he'd been keeping an eye on me, too, and could even name some random bloke I'd danced with but, at the time, he did a good impression of someone who, now that he knew I had played a joke on him, pretending to be French, was not remotely interested. It was such a shame.

Still, after a fun night, Alison and I got our coats and headed to the exit, wincing in our now painful high heels. Any discomfort in my feet, though, was immediately forgotten when, lo and behold, I saw a flash of lilac heading up the stairs in front of me – alerting me to Ash's back and his rather nice behind.

Thinking that I had nothing to lose, I promptly dashed up the stairs and bit him on the arse. Well, it seemed like a good idea at the time.

Ash jumped about ten foot in the air and then turned to stare at me, giving me a look that distinctly said, 'You're mental.' But then, the sides of his mouth began to twitch, and a laugh escaped. I giggled, too, and, in a few seconds flat, his frosty front had dispersed.

Ten minutes later, we were snogging in the car park.

'Will you be all right getting home?' he asked, stroking my hair, when we eventually came up for air. 'Do you want me to get you a taxi?'

He was such a sweetheart.

For some reason, I didn't take his number. I guess I just assumed we'd bump into each other again. I now had a very good reason to keep coming back to Tunbridge Wells!

And, as fate would have it, a few weeks later, I was in a bar with Alison when I spotted a familiar face.

Rather embarrassingly, I was wearing the same ravishing River Island suit (I was still strapped for cash and it was virtually my only going-out outfit) but, although Ash laughed about it, it didn't bother him at all, which made me like him even more.

I really fancied him. He was everything I'd never had in a boyfriend. Yes, he had that manly thing going on, but I could tell he also had a really smart and sensitive side to his character. He was the sort of person who just kept on surprising you.

Alison and I spent the whole night with him and his friends, and we headed to Da Vinci's again, where I tried, unsuccessfully, to get Ash to dance.

Later, we went back to Alison's parents' place for a nightcap.

Bless Alison – she soon made herself scarce so Ash and I

could spend some time alone. But, although we both knew we were very attracted to one another, it wasn't just about that. We sat and drank tea and talked for hours. In fact, we couldn't stop talking.

Before Ash left, we exchanged numbers and arranged our first date. It was two weeks away, and Ash wanted to take me for dinner.

I said goodbye and headed to bed with butterflies in my tummy, feeling happy and elated. After that, I thought about him all day every day.

By the time the day of our date finally arrived, I could hardly contain myself. I was so excited.

I got ready at Alison's and, now that I look back, my outfit was as horrendous as the red power suit. This time, I wore skintight black stirrup ski pants, with a white jacket (with shoulder pads, of course) and lots of red lipstick.

'You look lovely,' my suitor declared when he saw me. Bless him, he always has been good at saying what I want to hear. And there's no accounting for taste!

Ash took me to a beautiful Indian restaurant, which we still go to now, and it was just amazing. Our conversation was flirty and full of wind-ups and one-upmanship. That's what we were like (what we are still like), always playing games, being cool, but ultimately being really adoring with each other. The connection has always been deep, and Ash has always known exactly how to deal with me, right from the beginning.

As the weeks went by and we saw each other regularly, I loved spending time with him. Everyone does. He is so charismatic, the loveliest guy, and people just gravitate towards him. It was so easy, being with him – we'd just sit, have a bottle of wine and a chat. The hours would evaporate when we were talking. Quite simply, I fell head over heels in love with him, and I could tell he was smitten with me too. Girls just know these things!

In the many years that followed, the time that led us to this point – finally settling down and having Gigi – we've had our ups and downs, and lots of them. We've gone our separate ways more times than I care to remember, only to reconcile and start all over again, our paths always inextricably linked. I believe in fate, and I know that we are meant to be together.

Through all the highs and lows, one thing we've always done is talked.

Even now, sixteen years into our relationship, we'll go to bed – even if it's the early hours – and cuddle up together and have a chat. I love our little chats. They have been key to our relationship from day one.

From the first moment I met Ash, I also realized how bright he was. He's got a real thirst for knowledge, is a natural story-teller and is very well read. His general knowledge is fantastic, and he's always reeling off facts, teaching me about the Roman emperors or all the capital cities of the world or something. I love him telling me stuff, and he loves teaching me.

Although we hit it off straight away, however, it was years before we committed to each other or took the plunge and moved in together. In truth, I was always raring to just go for it, but Ash was more cautious.

Although I was younger than he was, not even in my twenties when we first met, it was me who wanted to settle down. Ash already had a few serious relationships under his belt and had been badly burnt. He felt he still had to lead his own life for a while, and was holding back, wanting to take things slowly. It was always me pushing him, tapping away for commitment, and him refusing to be bamboozled, procrastinating rather than progressing, taking his time and moving step by careful step. He nearly drove me round the bend!

Having said that, Ash has always been very caring and did start to look after me, almost immediately I met him.

Maybe because he was seven years older than I was, he was more worldly wise, so he was always encouraging me and thinking about what was best for me. There was also the fact that my family lived 400 miles away, so he was my support network, always giving me good advice, and always pushing me with my career.

When I first met him, I was out of work, so he'd constantly be on my case, asking me what auditions I'd been to, whether I'd been proactive about getting work that day, as I had said I would.

Over the years, Ash has never once let me feel sorry for myself; he's just got an indestructible spirit. Being with him often make me feel like I'm Rocky Balboa, and Ash is giving me the pep talk, psyching me up for a fight. Even, years later, when I felt at my absolute lowest ebb, during the chemotherapy, he was always there, giving me that vital boost. When all I wanted to do was wallow in self-pity, feeling battered and broken, he was the one lifting me up off the floor and encouraging me to fight another day. He's great for me like that.

Right from those early days, Ash helped to spark a real inner confidence in me, which I hadn't really had since I'd gone to drama college.

I made up my mind that I wanted to go to stage school at an early age.

I first auditioned at the age of eleven in the hope that I could get a scholarship for the Royal Ballet School in Richmond, Surrey. Although I didn't get in, they sent me a kind rejection letter, which said I did have talent and shouldn't give up. After that, I was determined not to.

I had my heart set on the famous Sylvia Young Theatre School, but it was based in Marylebone, London, 400 miles away from my home in Torquay. I was barely a teenager at the time and, if I won a place, it would mean having to stay with a family in London, something Mum didn't feel comfortable with.

Instead, I carried on going to the Pamela de Waal School

of Dancing in Torbay, which I'd attended since the age of three.

As I grew older, my passion for performing grew too, but times were hard. When I was fifteen, my parents had an acrimonious break-up and divorced, which meant that Mum, who'd always been instrumental in encouraging me in my dancing and acting, was now strapped for cash.

A year later, when I was invited for an interview at the prestigious Doreen Bird College of Performing Arts in Sidcup, I knew it was my big chance. If I got a place there, Mum would need to find £100 for the joining fee, but then, hopefully, a grant from the local education authority would fund the rest.

I put a lot of pressure on myself – the level of talent there was very high – but there was no question of me not getting in. Performing was my life, but I knew I couldn't expect my parents to pay.

On the day of my interview, Mum and I travelled up from Devon, both of us nervous and excited.

To win a place at the school, applicants had to prove they had what it took by participating in a number of classes, performing a piece of drama and a piece of dance, and to do well in a grilling in front of an interview panel.

When we arrived, I quickly changed into my pale-blue unitard (a delightful skin-tight one-piece garment with built-in leggings that went down to my feet) and my prized red jazz boots, which I just loved.

My first test was to take part in ballet and jazz modern classes. I did my best, but the standard was high. Then I had to perform a solo dance and a song in front of the panel of teachers, and follow it with some acting. I'd written a character piece about my parents getting divorced for my GCSE drama exam and, after agonizing about it for weeks, I decided to go with that, hoping it would meet with the panel's approval. It was a risk performing something unknown but, after I had done it, I thought they seemed reasonably impressed. But what was it they were scribbling on their notepads? Had I passed the test?

Finally, there was an interview and, by this point, like me, I could tell Mum was feeling the strain. For twenty minutes, the principal and various teachers fired questions at me and Mum, then they asked me who I most admired.

'Joan Collins!' I blurted out, right off the bat.

It seemed like an obvious answer. I'd been transfixed by *Dynasty* as a kid, and I've never been afraid of a bit of glamour. I loved it.

In fact, even if, for a lot of the past year, I may have slobbed around in a tracksuit, with no hair and no eyelashes, I've always had a bit of gloss on. Thank you, Joan Collins!

But when I said her name at the interview, they laughed at me. Perhaps they thought it was a strange answer for your average sixteen-year-old to give. I began to worry that I'd messed everything up.

Soon, though, the agony was over. I nearly whooped for joy when they offered me a place. Then poor Mum duly got out her chequebook and coughed up £100 then and there. We were both so chuffed. We'd done it!

I'd grown up loving the film *Fame* and, on my way out from the audition, I peeked into the commonroom and caught my first glimpse of that environment for real. My eyes darted around the room, and I saw loads of cool, extrovert people hanging around, looking like every one of them could steal a leading role in the movie.

All the girls were wearing matching navy-blue leotards with pink tights and had their hair in buns. They seemed so confident and beautiful. Some were holding court, peppering what they were saying with big, flamboyant arm gestures; others were raising their hands to the ceiling in graceful stretches; and one or two were just sitting still, script pages perched on their laps, lost in studying their lines. Every one of them looked so laidback and self-assured. I couldn't wait to be one of those girls.

Then, before I knew it, I was!

I found digs with a nice family called the Pinders, although, as ever with me, my introduction to life there was a comedy moment that involved me walking dog poo in on my shoes and all over their fabulous carpet! After this hilarious, if slightly embarrassing, start to life in my new home, I had no trouble settling into college and made lots of really great friends. We all wanted the same thing, so it was easy to bond and, soon, I was one of a gaggle of very noisy girls.

I was actually terribly shy in social situations so, as a cover-up, I quickly assumed the role of the mouthy, comedic one. I would hum all the way through drama classes to get a cheap laugh and put Olbas Oil in my eyes to turn myself into a weeping, red-eyed hag while singing 'Memories'.

It sounds disruptive, but it was really a distraction from the fact that I felt out of my depth and spent the whole time worrying that I wasn't good enough and didn't deserve to be at the college. We'd often throw parties and would be up dancing all night, but it was all very innocent fun. I didn't smoke more than anyone else whilst I was there, and I've never been able to drink loads. I'd invariably have a few glasses then be sick, so I didn't bother after a while. I was more than happy with a cup of tea and biccies.

Pretty much all of the three years I spent at college were an utter joy. Every day, we laughed, we played pranks, we cried, and ultimately, we worked very hard. We'd live in each other's pockets all week then go off to someone's hometown every weekend.

One week we'd all get the coach up to Lincolnshire, the next we'd go to Norfolk. We'd seek out the best dance clubs in London or drive to a nightclub in Norwich called Hollywood's (how apt) on a Monday, dance all night and then get up for an eight o'clock ballet class the next day.

The girls who attended our college were a talented lot – we had Melanie C. from the Spice Girls, for example, and a few other brilliant girls who went on to achieve great success in their own chosen areas.

As well as learning lots about performing, another thing all that training helped instil in me was a sense of discipline, which has stayed with me throughout my life. I haven't been late for a single medical appointment – chemo, radiotherapy or whatever. I pride myself on punctuality, and that has a great deal to do with my time at college.

I loved those years – but there was one dampener, a teacher who left me seriously doubting myself.

As part of our course, we'd go to primary schools in local areas and perform for the children. I adored it and put everything into it. One particular day, we were acting out some of Aesop's fables, and I was the narrator. Suddenly, one of the girls in the cast froze. I looked up and caught her eye; she looked petrified. It left us with no choice but to improvise. Once I'd had more stage experience, I realized that these things do happen but, at that moment, it was terrifying. Our teacher was furious and clearly seemed to think that, as I was the narrator and therefore linking the piece, it was all my fault. Afterwards, she laid into me in front of the whole class. I was devastated.

'Rebekah Gibbs, you are completely unprofessional,' she spat. 'You might as well give up now, you'll never work as an actress. You are a disgrace.'

I cannot tell you how gutted I was. It was a proper Simon Cowell-style slating. Yes, I may have been the class clown, but I'd worked so hard on that module and, in five seconds flat, she'd destroyed my dreams.

I looked at her, tears in my eyes, and went home to cry. I was inconsolable that night. Bless my landlady at the time, Mrs Robinson – she was so worried about me that she called up my mum; but nothing anyone could say could raise my spirits. If only I'd had Ash around back then! I knew I'd done nothing wrong, but it floored me to be on the receiving end of such unfair criticism.

Although I eventually picked myself up and decided to prove that tutor wrong, my confidence had taken a real pounding.

I left Doreen Bird with good marks and landed my part in the *Rocky Horror Picture Show*, but that one teacher's words were always ringing in my ears. With each job I got, slowly and surely I began to believe in myself, but it did take a bit of time.

Ash, however, had a real knack of giving me a boost. Within weeks of us first meeting, he'd made it his mission to encourage me.

'You'll be all right, you will,' he always told me. 'I have a good feeling about you.'

And he said it with such conviction that even I believed him!

He was right, too: I did land a brilliant part – in the newly created stage show of *Copacabana*. I felt one step closer to my goal – I was in a West End show. What better way for me to get some experience?

I was so excited, but there was one problem. Taking the part meant going off on tour first and hardly seeing Ash at all. I was torn, overjoyed to be in work again, doing what I totally adored, but also worried because of Ash and our future together.

Ash worked as a managing director, running the family business, an accident repair centre, and he worked ridiculously hard (he still does!). There was no way he would be able to take time off in the week to see me, and even the weekends would be a struggle.

We discussed our options, but there was no doubt about it: finding time to see each other was going to be tough. Could we really cope with snatched moments together once or twice a month?

'I can't do it, Beck,' Ash told me sadly. 'We've been spending all this time together, and now I won't see you for months. You need to go and do this on your own.'

I could tell by looking at his face he couldn't be swayed. I was too proud to cry in front of him, so I went home and sobbed into my pillow. Although I'd never told him, I loved him (it was a girly pride thing, and he knew anyway!), and splitting up with him was heartbreaking.

It was to be the first of many break-ups instigated by each of us over time. My work made our relationship like a tug-of-war: in between shows we'd inevitably get back together, but then I'd get called off again and we'd go our separate ways, neither one of us sure how best to make things work.

Ash never once asked me not to go on tour, and I never once offered to stay behind. Although we both really wanted to be together, our lives were out of sync, and neither of us was willing to compromise. It just wasn't an option for Ash to have a long-distance relationship, and I'd never pass up an opportunity to perform – it would go against all the hard work I'd been putting in since I first started performing, aged three. Be it right or wrong, I'd always made sacrifices for work. It was just par for the course.

The first time I realized that my all-consuming love of dancing came at a price was when I was about eight years old. It was a boiling-hot summer's day and I was sitting in a sweltering classroom trying hard to concentrate, my skin clammy and irritated from the heat, when my friend Caroline Daniels leant forward over her desk and whispered to me.

'Do you want to come swimming in my grandma's pool after school?' she asked.

'Yeah!' I blurted, without a moment's hesitation.

I'd been to Caroline's grandma's pool before, and it was ace. All afternoon, I kept imagining the lovely cool water and how we'd have so much fun, running and jumping and splashing about. Her grandma always made nice sandwiches, too, and, once you'd gobbled those up, she had a really long, exciting garden to explore. I couldn't wait. As soon as the bell sounded for the end of school, I grabbed my bag and pegged it back home.

Running through the back door, I saw my mother and immediately spluttered, 'Mummy, Mummy, Caroline has invited me to go swimming!'

But, rather than sharing my enthusiasm, she just looked at me with a really straight face.

'Well, Rebekah,' she said. 'You have to make your mind up – are you going swimming or to your ballet lesson?'

Groaning, I threw down my bag, remembering it was a dancing night. The last thing I wanted to do was to go to ballet in this heat, but I knew I couldn't miss a class to go swimming.

In that moment, I caught a glimpse of the future. I knew I had to decide what was more important. I thought: Mum and Dad spend all that money on my ballet, and it's what I want to do. I'm going to have to sacrifice lovely things like going swimming on a beautiful summer's day. Not even the temptation of Caroline's granny's pool was going to stop me going to ballet!

I'd always known I'd be in for a life in entertainment, as I'd started dancing at the age of three to help me beat the bulge – quite a comedy way to start, I think!

Mum had taken me to the doctor's and because I was

knock-kneed, clinically obese and lazy, dancing seemed like the perfect solution. I never looked back!

I loved my ballet lessons, especially the imaginary side of things and, before long, I was skipping along to classes every Monday evening. My parents both worked, my mum Anne as a secretary and my dad Ron as a builder, but they were far from rolling in it, so I had to convince them early on that I was serious about dancing and acting, and that the investment was worth all the hard-earned cash they were putting into it.

I was competitive, too, which is just as well, as I've never been one of those people who is just naturally good at everything without needing to try. I have always had to work hard, and I always refused to give up if I had a knockback. If there was an obstacle in my way, I would just keep on plugging away until I got to where I wanted to be.

In later years, I had to adopt the same attitude to fight my breast cancer. There has never been even a chance that I was going to allow the Big C to win – there is too much at stake, and there's nothing I love more than a good fight!

I can remember being five years old and feeling really cross when I only came fourth in my first performing-arts festival, with an acting and dancing piece. I was absolutely mortified that another little girl, called Rebecca, too, had scooped the top prize.

With the annual ballet competition coming up a few weeks later, I was determined to be the winner. I had started competing properly after my mum had finally given in and let me loose on the performance circuit. Now, like some kind of devil child, I paced the house, telling Mum, 'I'm going to win that competition.'

There I was, practising in my little pink tutu, ballet shoes and pink socks, with pink flowers in my hair, looking all cute and like butter wouldn't melt, when, in fact, underneath it all, I was getting stuck into some hardcore Noel Edmonds-style cosmic ordering – envisaging how exactly I was going to win!

Anyway, sure enough, the ballet festival competition came, I did my dancing – and I won it!

I always knew I'd have to try and try and keep knocking on doors until, eventually, one would open. And, even then, when opportunities arose, I'd have to make sacrifices to be able to take them and make the most of them.

When I made that decision to turn down swimming for my ballet class at the age of eight, I set the standard for the next fifteen years pretty much. In the years to come I would sacrifice spending time with Ash, and I would sacrifice home life, and birthdays, funerals and weddings.

There was so much I just couldn't make it to. Even when I first started *Casualty*, I missed the funeral of a very dear family friend, as well as Ash's sister's wedding. I just wasn't in a position to ask for time off.

I think that perhaps Ash got used to this over time but, back when we first met, us having a long-distance relationship just wasn't something he felt he could do. He wasn't about to let his heart rule his head so, reluctantly, we went our separate ways. I headed off to take my part in *Copacabana*.

Despite the upset of splitting up with Ash, being on tour was the perfect distraction. With the excitement of the show, I couldn't be miserable for long, not when I was working on a live show that was a laugh a minute.

To my delight, my twenty-first birthday coincided with our first preview in Plymouth. And what a celebration it was. After the show, I was thrilled when the whole cast piled into the the Bank, a pub behind the theatre. Even the creative team was there, including, to my great delight, Barry Manilow. I couldn't believe that I was in the same room as BM! They all sang a special version of 'Happy Birthday', including Barry, and I was given a cake and some gorgeous perfume. We went on to party until the early hours of the morning. I was the last one standing! What a twenty-first birthday to remember – I was living my dream, surrounded by my friends and in the same room as my childhood hero. Life didn't get any better than this.

The tour went on, and it was a real riot. Often I'd find myself thinking, I can't wait to tell Ash about this!, then I'd get that sinking feeling when I remembered we weren't together any more. I couldn't call him and fill him in all those little comedy moments I knew he would find hilarious. Ash and I have always shared a wacky, slightly mental sense of humour and, when we weren't together, I missed being able to laugh with him. In fact, I missed everything about him, about us. But I also tried to be philosophical, telling myself that if our not being together was what he wanted, I had to respect that. One of the things I have always found so attractive (and infuriating!) about Ash is that he totally knows his own mind. He won't be swayed – and our daughter is exactly the same!

That period, when I was in *Copacabana*, turned out to be one of the longest times Ash and I didn't speak. It was difficult and depressing being apart from Ash, even though I was doing exactly what I'd always wanted to and loving my job. I have since discovered (after a wave of questioning when we did get back together) that Ash felt as lost and miserable as I did.

As the months went by, being apart from Ash didn't really get any easier. I was twenty-one and living out of a bag, and in limbo emotionally. I'd spend weekends on tour and go out to all the clubs with my friends from the cast, all the time trying desperately not to think about Ash.

The thing is, he'd knocked me for six; I just couldn't get him out my head. I found myself wondering if there was more to life than endless partying.

I thought back to the boyfriends I'd had before. One of them was the actor Jude Law, who'd been my on-off teenage sweetheart for a couple of years when we were both appearing in National Youth Music Theatre productions.

At the age of fifteen, we'd spent time together at the Edinburgh Fringe Festival, and I'd been enthralled by him. Before he even asked me out I was so excited at the thought of him being in the dormitory downstairs that I could hardly eat!

Anyway, we did eventually kiss, and he was just glorious. He was the first boy ever to take me on a date. Because I had been performing from such a young age and had become fixated on being the best, I had missed out on a lot of 'normal' life. When everyone else was messing around climbing trees and riding their bikes in big groups of mates, I was madly practising ballet and tap, which didn't leave much time for anything else. As a result, I had very little confidence around boys. But something clicked when I hit fifteen, I suddenly felt intrigued by the opposite sex, and when I met Jude, it all came together for me. I thought he was gorgeous.

We were only fifteen and living away from our parents, and there were strict rules, so we had to sneak out to meet up for our date. I had to creep down to his dorm after curfew, and then the pair of us climbed through the window and made our escape.

As we ran down the street, Edinburgh was buzzing with life because of the festival, but we managed to find the one Chinese restaurant with not a soul in it. I didn't care, though, I was so excited to be out on my first date.

Jude smoked Marlboro and seemed very grown up. He was great fun to be around.

On my opening night, he got me this silver aquamarine bangle. He'd searched the length and breadth of Edinburgh to find a box to put it in. He had star quality and style even then – aged fifteen!

After Jude, I dated a guy called Simon, who was a dancer. I was eighteen and he was twenty-four. He didn't do dinner dates. I guess he didn't have much money. We went for one meal in the year we were together, and I paid!

After him, I really wanted to find myself a gentleman and, finally, I'd met one. Ash blew Simon, and even Jude, out of the water in the chivalry stakes. When we were apart, I tormented myself, wondering whether I had done the right thing to have let a man like him slip through my fingers.

I cried myself to sleep sometimes, but what could I do? I'd made my choice. I'd worked so hard to get to where I was, and I couldn't give that up now, no matter how much it hurt. Then my pride would kick in and I'd remind myself that he wasn't exactly giving up anything for me either!

In June 1994, *Copacabana* moved to the Prince of Wales Theatre in London. Our opening night was delayed, as they had to re-work the set. One good thing about the delay, though, was that it gave me time to find somewhere to live, with my friend Kerry, another dancer from the show.

We quickly found ourselves a lovely little place in West Hampstead (well, it was more Kilburn really, but West Hampstead sounded posher), we moved in and immediately made it our own, all cosy and warm. I loved that flat – we called it our Peach Palace – and nothing was more comforting than the two of us getting home, changing into our pyjamas and curling up on the sofa with a cup of tea to chat. It felt like home right away.

But, as content as I was, there was still a feeling of emptiness deep inside me. Something – or rather, someone – was missing.

My new flat was miles away from Ash's stomping ground in Tunbridge Wells, but I just couldn't stop thinking about him. One night, after the show, I rang him up on a whim, butterflies in my tummy. It had been six months since we'd last spoken.

'Hello?' he croaked sleepily.

'Hiya,' I said nervously. 'Did I wake you? I just thought I'd call – for a chat really.'

'That's weird,' he replied. 'I've just been dreaming about you.'

We've always been very in tune with each other like that and, straight off, we were chatting away. It was as if no time at all had passed since we had last talked.

Well, that was that. Ash came to see the show a few nights later and, afterwards, I went to meet him at the stage door.

'You were wonderful, Rebekah,' he said, greeting me with a grin. He looked like he'd burst with pride. Him feeling that way made my eyes well up and, when he gave me a big hug, it just felt so right. Immediately, we were back on again, and this time it was better than ever.

Often, Ash would come to London and we'd spend the entire weekend together, just talking and doing nice stuff – going sightseeing, for walks by the Thames or for lovely meals out. It was heavenly. I knew I was head over heels in love with him and had been for a long time, but nothing had ever been said. I was waiting for him to say it first. I'm old-fashioned like that.

One weekend, we were sitting on the floor together, just before Ash had to leave to drive back to Tunbridge Wells. I could tell there was something on his mind.

Putting his hand to my face, he stroked my cheek. 'I love you, Rebekah,' he told me, looking deep into my eyes. He said it in such an earnest and deep-felt way that it just took my breath away.

And I immediately said it back.

After that, we were always telling each other. There's nothing nicer than that feeling of being totally in love and knowing it is reciprocated. Life was great. We saw each other all the time and were nauseatingly happy.

For my twenty-second birthday, Ash picked me up from the show and drove me back to his place. When we arrived in Tunbridge, he had a surprise for me.

'See that car there, sweetheart?' he said, pointing to a red Fiat Uno. 'It belongs to you.'

He'd even written 'Becks' on the back. No one had ever done anything like that for me before, and I couldn't believe it.

I named my new set of wheels Victoria (as you do with your first car). Having a car gave me a lot of freedom. Now I could drive home to Devon to see my family and, most weekends, I'd jump in and head off on the M25 to see Ash. We'd spend the weekend hanging out at his home or driving round the Kent countryside, fantasizing about buying the beautiful houses we'd pass.

Another blissful year followed, with me attempting to carve out a career with *Copacabana* and eventually earning my stripes as an understudy. Ash encouraged me all the way.

As the end of the show approached, I was concerned I'd be out of work, but I needn't have worried: next, I landed a part on tour with Jim Davidson.

It was September 1996, and I was one third of a three-piece singing group on the road with the lovely JD. Suddenly, I'd upped my wages, and we went touring around Ireland, Germany and Holland, entertaining the troops. I'd been apprehensive about being away for a few months but, by this point, Ash seemed to have got his head round it. One small step for man . . . but it was a different story when I got back and asked him to move in with me!

My flatmate, Kerry, was getting married, so it was time to bid goodbye to the Peach Palace and find somewhere else to live. I tried my hardest to persuade Ash, but he told me time and again that he didn't feel the time was right for us to move in together. Reluctantly, I found a place in Wimbledon with three other girls, and channelled all my energy into work. I was cross and upset that I couldn't control everything to do with my and Ash's relationship – it seemed so natural to me that we should move on to the next stage. It didn't ever occur to me that I was missing out on being young and crazy like others in the cast were – I just didn't want that.

While I was on tour with Jim, my agent had rung to say that my dream job had come in: a role in *Starlight Express*! Every theatre actress has her three ultimate shows, and *Starlight Express* was right up there for me. When I heard that David Grimrod was putting a cast together, I set my sights on being part of it. To prepare for the auditions, a big group of hopefuls had to endure months of skating school.

Skating school? – it was more like a full-on boot camp!

I thought I was a dead cert, after skate school the final audition had gone brilliantly and I was sure that I was definitely in. I remember taking the call and being all geared up to have the 'I hope you can start rehearsing in January' conversation (I already had it blocked out in my new diary). I waited and waited for that call and, when it came, it was David Grimrod himself phoning me. I was so nervous answering, anticipating that all my dreams were about to come true. Instead, David uttered the simple words: 'You haven't got it, darling, it didn't work out this time.' I thought, What the f**k do you mean, It didn't work out? I'm perfect for your show!

I like to think I'm a realist, and I do believe that, as an actress, you intrinsically know what you are right and wrong for. But it was funny – even though I'd just been turned down, I didn't think, Right, that's it, I'll never do *Starlight Express*; I just felt my time would come. And, sure enough, three months later, it did. Someone dropped out, and I was cast as their replacement. I was so elated when I got that call (I'm sure I must have pierced David's eardrum with my manic screaming!). I trained and trained – getting prepared for my dream role took over my life.

Learning how to perform on skates, eight hours a day, was every bit as gruelling as you'd imagine, and every inch of my body was in pain. In fact, the crippling three-month course of chemo I went on to endure years later is about the only thing I've ever known that could top that feeling of achiness and fatigue.

Every day, I'd sing, dance and fall on my arse, over and over again. It was tough, but brilliant. The day of the final dress rehearsal, they asked the choreographer Arlene Phillips, who is now best known as a judge on *Strictly Come Dancing*, to give us feedback on our performance. She's always been a razor-tongued taskmaster and, back then, we waited anxiously for her verdict.

'I have one piece of advice for all the girls,' she said coolly. 'You all need to go to the gym!' Ouch! It sounded harsh at the time but, the thing about Arlene is that she wants you to be the best you possibly can be.

I've never been so nervous as on that opening night. It was abject fear. Most opening nights, I did wonder why on earth I was putting myself through all this, but then the adrenalin would kick in and suddenly I'd be reminded of how much I loved it. The rush of euphoria when we pulled off our first *Starlight* show was amazing. I wish I could have bottled that feeling.

In the end, I did two years on *Starlight* in the West End. I'd never been fitter! There was no room for partying – I'd get off stage and I'd be home and in bed by 11 p.m.

After *Starlight*, I went straight into another job at the New London Theatre. I was having a great run of London shows, Ash and I had been together three years, and everything was looking rosy.

I'd been wearing Ash's resistance to our moving in together down over time and, after lots of me sulking and using emotional blackmail, he'd at last agreed to let me move into his bachelor pad in Tunbridge. I felt it was a momentous achievement.

As soon as he'd given me the go-ahead, I arrived in my little Fiat, Victoria, grinning from ear to ear and laden with boxes of my junk. For Ash, on the other hand, adjusting to me moving in definitely took a bit of getting used to.

His home was very much his pride and joy – you had to take your shoes off before you were even allowed over the threshold. Things were quite strained between us at first. We were always having our little spats, as I think most couples do when they first move in together. He'd leave all the dirty washing to pile up and then do it in one big purge, while I preferred to do it as I went along. He accused me of 'stealing' his drawers, so I'd ask if he really did need to fill them with about a thousand old, yellowing receipts and a mountain of golf tees. (Thank God we don't have that problem now; we built Ash an extension on the house specifically for him to put all his tat in!) After a while, though, we both calmed down and we began to iron out the creases. Then it was lovely and we settled into domestic bliss.

I loved living with Ash. It made things so much easier, and we'd finally made a real commitment.

Every night, we'd drift off to sleep side by side. I felt content, happy and secure. But I was still ambitious.

Starring in *Grease* had always been one of my ultimate aims. I heard rumours from my agent that there would be casting for a new production, so I made some phone calls and then spoke to my agent – I wasn't prepared to leave anything to chance. At the time I was doing a singing gig at the New London theatre – what's known in the business as a 'fill in'. I'd heard the girls excitedly talking about going for the role of Rizzo, or Sandra Dee and all the rest. I joined in, well aware that this was one of the big ones.

Once I'd secured my audition, I went into overdrive – I was going for Rizzo. On the day, I arrived nearly two hours early to 'get in the zone'. It's so important to do this – you've got to feel that inner confidence tingling through your body when you walk into the audition room. I ignored all the other girls waiting – I just didn't feel in the mood for chitchat; I really wanted to nail the part, so I had to concentrate. When my turn came around it all came together for me, and all my hard work paid off when I was told on the spot that I was good enough for the lead rather than starting as the understudy. I was sent home to prepare for my recall audition, well aware that I didn't have it in the bag quite yet. I bought the *Grease* soundtrack and listened to it on a loop; I even had the headphones on when I went to bed. I broke down every single line of that soundtrack and lived and breathed it.

I went back for my recall and was told I had the job. I'd got the role of Rizzo! It was the first time I'd bagged a starring role in a musical, and it was in *Grease*!

Oh my God, I'd loved *Grease* as a teenager. My oldest friend, Jane, and I would constantly stick the album on, pouting and crooning along to 'Look At Me, I'm Sandra Deee . . .'

It was such an opportunity, but I was worried how Ash

would take it. Being in *Grease* meant months on the road, away from him. My touring had split us up before, and I'd just fought long and hard to move in with him. How would he take it now, me running off again?

But, as hard as it must have been for him, Ash didn't stand in my way. He knew how important it was for me.

'It's your job, Becks,' he told me. 'We'll just have to find a way to make it work.'

Relieved, I packed up my stuff and headed off again.

This time, I was on the road for nearly eighteen months, and the venues ranged from as near as Eastbourne to as far away as Aberdeen. Ash and I saw each other whenever we could, but it was inevitable that my being on tour would put a distance between us. Although we talked on the phone all the time, the cast around me kind of became my family too. When I needed support, they were there for me, particularly when my grandma back in Devon passed away. Being on tour meant I hadn't been able to get back to see her as often as I'd have liked, and that haunted me. Being on stage seems, and is, glamorous, but boy do you have to make some tough sacrifices.

Whenever Ash came to visit or I went home for a day or two, it was as if we hadn't been apart. We'd be back winding each other up, having our chats and cuddles in front of the telly. But, each time I had to say goodbye again, it was torture, and I'd struggle not to cry.

In some ways, I suppose, it was easier for me. I was away

having fun, constantly going to new places, seeing new sights, while Ash was at home with my belongings all around, painfully aware that I wasn't there.

Not that he sat at home moping, he was living his own life, but I think he did focus on the light at the end of the tunnel – on the time when the tour would come to an end and I'd be back home.

Just as we were both counting down the days, my agent rang me. I'd been called for another audition, the lead role in *Fame*.

This was it, everything I had been building up to – I was auditioning for the role of Carmen, the confident but slightly cocky dancer with a big voice. There was one particular song that was massive, full of high notes, and I spent hours and days practising it. I knew that, ideally, they would be looking for a girl aged between fifteen and nineteen – I was nearly twenty-seven, so I was already at a disadvantage before I'd even started.

On the day of the audition I travelled from Milton Keynes to London, I arrived early, as usual, and went into my own little world. There were three of us going for the role, and we were all put in the green room together. I heard the other two girls practising in there, and I was devastated – they were amazing, *and* younger than I was. I was sure I stood no chance. Then my name was called and that something just kicked in again – I went in there to win, and I did. I got the job! But it meant another tour.

Again, I'd grown up listening to and watching *Fame* – and now I got to play Carmen, making my entrance on stage on top of a yellow taxi and singing the title song. It was too good to be true but, at the same time, it was heartbreaking. I knew that, as far as Ash was concerned, we couldn't survive another long stint apart. I had pushed him to the limit with my time on tour with *Grease*. He wouldn't put up with my absence indefinitely, and I couldn't blame him for that. I knew how being on the road affected my feelings too. It was so hard to keep it all going.

'I think it's time to call it a day,' Ash told me gently. I couldn't help but weep. He looked as if he was going to cry, too, but he was keeping it together, always proud, always stoic.

Our break-up wasn't at all explosive; there was no screaming or shouting or door-slamming. The two of us just sat there quietly, empty, knowing that, sometimes, no matter how much you love each other, the elements are against you.

Ash couldn't handle another tour, but he didn't want me to give up such a golden opportunity either, so he was letting me go. We'd tried to make it work for six years, but it was just too hard. It had to end.

'We'll still be best friends, Beck,' he said. 'If you ever need me, I'm only a phone call away.'

In one last act of thoughtfulness, he packed up all my stuff and drove to my mum's in Devon with it while I was away on tour. That's how amicable our break-up was, which made it all the more heartbreaking.

Those first few weeks after we split, I really struggled. I felt exhausted from crying, and emotionally stripped bare. If I was totally honest with myself, I resented him for giving up on us but, with that, was mixed up my own feelings of self-loathing and guilt that I'd put my career before my relationship.

But there was no way I could have turned my back on that opportunity. I knew there was a shelf life for doing this sort of thing and I didn't want to get to my thirties and still be on the road. That was when I wanted to settle down and have a family. I needed to fulfil my ambitions now and not live in regret later.

But what if I'd messed everything up? What if I'd lost the love of my life? I couldn't bear to think about it – so I didn't. I suppressed the heartbreak, and all my fears, and threw myself into my role as Carmen, giving it all I'd got.

The funny thing is that, now, Ash always says he's pleased that I went for it all guns blazing too. We've framed and hung lots of my pictures from those days but, when we look at the *Fame* ones, we both feel a little bit sad. Here are all these happy pictures and little messages from the cast, but it was at a time when Ash wasn't in my life. Looking back, I don't think it did me any harm. Having met Ash when I was so young, I did rely on him heavily, and having to stand on my own two feet was a good thing. That inner grit I had to find certainly stood me in good stead for what was to come. Whichever way you look at it, though, the reality is that we very nearly lost each other for good.

3. Sliding Doors

Watching Ash, always so worried and attentive, walk off to get me a glass of water, I took a deep breath and studied the toxic pink fluid which was pumping into my veins.

When you're sitting in hospital having chemotherapy, it gives you a lot of time to think. Time to contemplate those *Sliding Doors* moments, when your life could have taken a radically different route, changing your destiny for ever. Time to ponder on events and circumstances that sweep you up into unsuitable romances, and could so easily mean that you end up spending your life with someone else. In my case, that would mean a life without Ash supporting me now . . .

It was on a gorgeous spring day when I found myself at the top of the Eiffel Tower being proposed to by a devoted boyfriend.

Caught up in the romance of the stunning Paris scenery surrounding us, I immediately said yes. Why wouldn't I? He was down on one knee, he had the diamond ring and he loved me.

The date was 17 March, and it was my twenty-seventh birthday, but my husband-to-be wasn't Ash. He was actually called Lee and, in three months, he'd swept me off my feet.

When Ash and I broke up before my *Fame* tour, I found I hated being single but, at the same time, in many ways, I felt like giving up on love. I didn't have the energy or the inclination actively to go looking for romance, so when I met Lee, it just seemed so easy and comfortable.

I first got talking to him in the steamroom at the gym, of all places. I'd been relaxing in there before the show that evening and liked him instantly. He was just so easy to talk to, and I looked at him and thought how similar he was to Ash.

Like Ash, Lee was tall, he had the same build, and was about the same age – eight years older than me. I guess alarm bells should have started ringing then, but I was oblivious. I felt lonely, and I knew what I liked. If my tick list had all Ash's qualities on it, then what could I do?

Lee was a good man and, straight away, he wanted to look after me. I guess, being old-fashioned, that is always something I have gone for in a boyfriend. He was chivalrous and encouraging and committed to me very quickly. Even more importantly, he understood, and was prepared to fit in with, my job.

Lee told me he didn't believe in playing games and announced that he loved me within weeks.

Then, just a few months into our romance, he arranged

a trip to Paris for my birthday. We stayed in a beautiful hotel in the city centre and spent our time shopping, going for delicious meals and just sitting, watching the world go by.

On the afternoon of my birthday, Lee surprised me by saying he wanted to go up the Eiffel Tower. We went to a restaurant in the middle of the tower, which had amazing views. Lee was really scared of heights but, seeing as we were both a bit tiddly after having champagne and wine with our lunch, I assumed he was full of Dutch courage. But travelling up and up and up in the rickety lift, he began to look rather pale.

'Are you OK?' I asked, squeezing his arm. He smiled back, but he definitely looked more than a bit queasy.

Once we'd reached the top, Lee still looked really nervous, and it wasn't long before I discovered why. As I was admiring the Paris skyline, suddenly he touched my arm. Next, he produced a ring box and, *voilà!* I was his fiancée!

I waited for the rush of excitement to hit me, but it didn't come. Instead, within seconds of accepting, I started to get that little niggling feeling that I'd been too hasty.

I held his hand and beamed and examined my beautiful ring over and over but, on the way down in the lift, as I snuggled into his chest, thoughts were racing through my head. I started to persuade myself that the engagement was a good thing. I told myself that he was a nice guy, he was funny, he loved me, he'd look after me . . .

But in the fifteen minutes it took us to find a taxi to take us back to the hotel, I was beginning to have big doubts. It was such a massive thing, I thought, and he doesn't really know me and I don't know him.

Instinctively, my thoughts began to wander to Ash. The problem was, essentially, that Lee had a very tough act to follow.

If I thought back to the years I'd spent with Ash, there were so many lovely, meaningful memories. Ash had known me since I was nineteen. I'd grown up in those years, and we had so many shared experiences. And it wasn't just about memories – I knew deep down that how I felt with Ash was exactly how it was meant to feel – funny how you only really understand that when it's gone.

After a romantic couple of days, Lee and I flew back to the UK. I was living with him up North and, soon, word of our engagement was spreading like wildfire.

Now, after blowing hot and cold inside my head for days, I decided to bury any doubts. I'm quite stubborn like that. I knew I couldn't spend my life wondering 'what if' about Ash. After all, he'd had his chance – he'd been the one to decide it was over. 'This is my new life,' I told myself.

So I just got on with it. I was enjoying playing Carmen in *Fame*, and Lee was lovely. He knew the show was exhausting at times, so he'd do really thoughtful things, like buy me a lilo to sleep on between shows or turn up with a coffee to keep me going. He was great husband material.

I quickly became the girl of his family, who were incredibly welcoming. I made friends with his friends and went all out to be the devoted fiancée. I tried so hard to make it all fit together, but still it didn't quite feel right. Sometimes, I'd wake up crying in the morning and I'd have to conceal it. As I wept into my pillow, my fiancé sleeping, oblivious, I'm ashamed to say I was crying over Ash – how bad is that?

If Lee did wake up and ask me what was wrong, I'd have to try to cover it up.

'It was just a silly nightmare, honey,' I'd tell him, wiping my eyes and trying to smile. I couldn't believe what a mess I'd got myself into.

By now, I had no contact with Ash at all. He'd completely frozen me out, so I knew he'd heard my news. Of course, he wouldn't have expected me to be a wallflower – and he was certainly out meeting girls – but I knew the bombshell that I was marrying someone else would leave him devastated. I could only imagine how I would feel if the tables were turned – I'd want to kill him!

It hadn't taken long for him to find out. A friend of his came to see the show and spotted my engagement ring. I begged him not to say anything, saying I wanted to call Ash myself, but of course he went and told him straight away.

For days, I rang and rang Ash's phone, but he never picked up or called me back. I cried myself to sleep that whole week, I felt so cruel. Ash was still my best mate and

I couldn't bear the thought of him feeling like shit. I had so many things I wanted to say to him, but it was no good. In the end, I had to respect the fact he was getting on with things and I should just leave him be.

I think both us went into mourning at that point. It was just so permanent. It meant that Ash and I would never be together again. But he can't have cried any more than I did.

Almost immediately, Lee and I had set a date for the following year. He said he didn't want to wait around. Really, I should have found all this incredibly exciting and spontaneous but, although on the outside we may have seemed like the perfect couple in love, I was feeling more and more unsure. Looking back, Lee's need to hurry things along makes me certain he had a suspicion that all wasn't well. I would have done the same – it's as if you think marriage is the answer to everything when there are doubts, as if it fixes everything. In any case, and whether or not he'd guessed that I still had feelings for Ash, by Christmas I knew in my heart that I wasn't fooling anyone.

To this day, I don't know if Lee picked up on the real reason for my doubts, but I certainly felt his enthusiasm evaporate along with mine. We were planning the most important day of our lives, but neither of us could rustle up much enthusiasm for flowers, menus or wine-tasting. It was really sad, and I felt terrible about the whole thing – Lee was such a decent guy, and he loved me; his family were so warm, and he'd done nothing wrong. It was me who had the problem.

I couldn't help thinking back to when my parents got divorced. It had all been so hurtful. I'd never have been able to forgive myself for getting married knowing that I had doubts . . .

Lee and I had given it a good go. We really went for it but, that Christmas, we both expressed concern that things were running away from us. I guess he was worn down by my lack of enthusiasm. As much as he wanted to live the fairytale, even he had to admit defeat in the face of such a reluctant bride.

After a big heart to heart, we came to the difficult conclusion that there was something missing, and we'd been too hasty in getting engaged. We decided to call the wedding off, and broke up soon after.

As I'd suspected, I felt so relieved – it was like having a weight lifted from my shoulders. Straight away, I knew it was definitely the right decision, for both of us. Lee deserved to be with someone who adored him.

I moved back to London, bought my first flat and generally tried to keep my head down. I was just getting on with work and trying to avoid any more drama. I was trying to be a grown-up, standing on my own two feet.

Then the wedding day of my old pulling pal, Alison, arrived. She'd asked me to be bridesmaid, and it was all happening in a beautiful church in Tunbridge Wells.

Going back to Tunbridge Wells now I was no longer with Ash was weird. I felt like a stranger. I had that funny feeling in my tummy – half sick, half excited – as I passed all our old haunts: the restaurant Ash first took me to, the nightclub where we met, the places where we fell in love.

The church was just spellbinding, and Alison looked so gorgeous and happy. I was swept up in the romance of the day, and my thoughts turned to Ash. I'm going to marry Ash here, I smiled to myself, imagining my own walk down the aisle to greet my handsome groom.

Back to reality, Becks. No chance, I thought to myself, sadly.

The service was beautiful and, posing for photos with the bride and groom, I looked round at all the couples holding hands and gazing at each other adoringly in their lovely dresses and suits.

As I stood there, smiling happily, a little voice inside my head was niggling away.

'I want to be part of a couple,' it was saying. 'I want to be with Ash.'

Why couldn't I get him out of my head? In truth, I'd been thinking about Ash throughout my relationship with Lee, and even more so after the split.

I'd recently quizzed my Aunty Rachel, who was the most happily married person I knew, how she had known that Uncle Clive was The One.

'How *do* you know?' I'd asked. 'What do you look for?'

'Marry your best friend,' she'd said decisively.

I'd been hanging on her words ever since.

Well, after a couple of glasses of champagne, the little voice in my head had become a huge, nagging one, urging me to pick up the phone and call Ash.

Determined to strike while the iron was hot, I tiptoed across the lawn haphazardly, trying to avoid the heels of my dainty bridesmaid's shoes sinking into the turf. Once I'd found a secluded spot, I rummaged around in my bag for my mobile phone. I dialled Ash's number, praying that he would pick up.

He answered within a couple of rings.

'Becks!' he announced. I was relieved to hear that he seemed surprised but pleased to hear from me. To be honest, I was totally thrown that he had picked up at all – after all, he'd been ignoring me for ages. But, soon, all became clear.

After we'd chatted for a while, he admitted that he'd heard my engagement to Lee was off.

'I was sorry to hear that, Rebekah,' he told me graciously. Same old Ash – although it did explain the fact that he'd only let the phone ring three times!

'What are you doing today?' I suddenly asked him, hearing music in the background.

'Actually, I'm best man at a wedding. Do you remember John?'

'Really?' I laughed. 'Fancy that!'

It had to be a sign. Just hearing Ash's voice again told me all I needed to know – I had to see him.

Within weeks, we were back dating again. And, this time, there was no way anything would break us up.

Of course, everyone was astounded that we'd got back together, although no one gave us a hard time about it. I think the people who cared about us had always known we were meant for each other – even when we didn't know it ourselves!

This time, there was no doubt in either of our minds. By now, I was twenty-eight, and Ash was thirty-five. We'd both grown up and knew exactly what we wanted – to settle down and be together, this time for good.

We very quickly bought a lovely house in Tunbridge Wells and got on with life together. At last the timing was right for both of us. Ash had sown his wild oats, and I'd taken the decision to give up musical theatre for a while. Not only had the touring taken its toll on me and Ash, but I wanted to try and expand my CV by pursuing straighter theatre and TV. Even so, Ash still lived and worked in Tunbridge Wells, and I would have to go where the work was.

Our first test came when I landed a role in a comedy farce that involved a tour. I broke it to Ash tentatively, praying that it wouldn't set us back to square one.

'All jobs come to an end, Becks,' he told me, squeezing my hand. 'And when you come home, I'll be here waiting.'

And that was that. At last it was the real deal. We'd both learnt our lesson.

Over the years, it hasn't always been plain sailing, but I've come to realize that not being with Ash is like losing my right arm. We're rock solid, and I don't believe anyone else would stand by me and support me like he has. I could never be without him. Ash will have to put up with me for the rest of my life, whether it turns out to be luxuriously long or cruelly cut short. Death is going to have to take me away from him, because nothing else will.

Once we'd committed and bought our house, I knew we'd always be together. But, as much as we had an amazing future ahead of us, like all men, Ash needed a little helping hand in the commitment stakes.

As more years passed – now more than a decade since we'd first met – I had my sights set on another important prize: that ring on my finger!

Now that we have a beautiful daughter and a wedding date set, Ash tells me that, deep down, he always wanted those things too. But, as many guys do, he was always waiting for the right moment (and the balls!) to do the deed.

It became almost farcical. Over the years, many perfect moments came and went when I really thought that Ash might propose.

There was the Christmas in Thailand when we were both having full body massages, with the relaxing rustle of banana leaves and the sea lapping on the shore the only sounds.

'Becks,' Ash said, smiling, as my heart skipped a beat. He's sooo going to ask me! I thought. 'This is gorgeous, isn't it?'

Bah!

And don't even get me started on the time we were sitting, surrounded by orange trees, in our favourite bustling square in Marbella, eating paella and watching the world go by. Or the night on the pier in Cyprus when we cuddled up on a little bench under a pretty white canopy looking out to the bay as the most beautiful sunset played out before us.

Despite all these missed opportunities, I never used to get angry. I always had faith that he would do it one day. It was only after I'd finished my two-year stint playing Nina on *Casualty* in May 2006 that I started to get impatient. We'd known each other for fourteen years by then, and I was surer than ever that Ash would finally decide to make an honest woman of me during our summer holiday to Marbella. Despite the fact that Ash's parents have a place near by, we'd rented our own fabulous secluded villa and, every day, we'd play the happy couple, getting up, going to the gym together. Then I'd prepare lunch, and, afterwards, we'd have the pool to ourselves. The villa was also completely private, so we could walk round in the buff, with not a care in the world!

This is how it's supposed to be, I thought to myself as we lounged by the pool, completely relaxed in each other's company. Me and him together. It just works.

The holiday was so romantic that, every day, I was sure he'd get on with it and ask me. We even looked at a beautiful eternity ring in the window of a jeweller's.

'I'll have that, babe!' I said, only half joking.

'We'll come back,' he told me, winking. But we never did. Still, it was a lovely holiday, one of the best we'd had.

At the airport for the trip back home, however, Ash not proposing was playing on my mind.

I studied his tanned face as he handed the check-in girl our passports. He looked lovely, really handsome and relaxed after a blissful two weeks. But, if he hadn't thought to propose this time, when would he ever?

So, after we'd checked in our bags, I sat down with Ash and ordered us cups of tea.

'Can I say something to you?' I asked him, clutching my mug nervously.

'Sure, babe, anything,' he replied, not even looking up from his Wilbur Smith novel.

I bit the bullet.

'If you haven't asked me to get married to you by the end of this year, I'm going to move on,' I said. But, rather than being all moody about it, I said it softly, with a slight smile on my face.

Ash looked at me and laughed. 'Give over, Becks,' he scoffed good-naturedly.

But something must have registered because, after that, he kept bringing it up.

In August, we were sitting watching TV together when, out of the blue, Ash reminded me of what I'd said.

'You know what you said before about if I don't ask you to marry me?'

'Yes, babe,' I answered.

'Will you move on?' he enquired.

'I will, babes, I will move on,' I told him. 'If we can't do it by end of this year, I don't think we'll ever do it.'

Like before, Ash laughed, using humour to deflect the seriousness of the situation.

'You'll actually leave this house?' he challenged me.

'Yes,' I said, looking him right in the eye. Then I turned back to the television.

As the end of the year drew near, I noticed that Ash seemed to be off a lot having secret little meetings. It seemed my 'unexplosive ultimatum', as my friend Sue had called it, might just be sinking in.

'Babe, I'm just going to see John,' Ash would say, grabbing his car keys on a Saturday and heading out the door. Or 'Babe, going out for a bit of business.'

'OK, babe,' I'd call back, smiling to myself. I just knew then he was going to do it.

But, as the weeks passed, nothing!

By this point, I'd often catch Ash staring into space with a furrowed brow. I suspected that he was now agonizing over where and how to make the proposal so, again, I couldn't help but meddle. I knew what was coming, and I didn't want him stressing unnecessarily about the detail.

'Do you know what, babe?' I told him. 'This house has been a really happy house, and it's blessed for us. If you asked me here, I'd be really happy. There's no need for a big fuss.'

Sure enough, within a week, it happened, on 16 December.

I was snuggled up in bed in my pyjamas watching *X Factor* when Ash pointed to the white Christmas tree with sparkling fairy lights we had in the bedroom.

'Look at the top of the tree, Beck,' he said.

'Ooh, is there some choccy on it?' I grinned, looking up.

But, instead, there at the top, sparkling away, was a gold ring with a stunning solitaire diamond.

It was so beautiful, and I was completely speechless. It was one of those surreal moments. I was just so shocked that it had actually happened after all these years.

'Oh, Ash!' I cried, my voice wobbling. I threw my arms round him.

Once I'd got over the shock – and accepted, of course! – we made love. Then we ordered a Chinese takeout to celebrate.

As far as I was concerned, it couldn't have been more romantic.

When I thought back to my time with Lee in Paris, I realized how all the grand gestures in the world couldn't have competed with Ash's proposal. It just suited me. It was Christmas time, it was cosy and lovely, and it was at home, one of my most special places.

I found out later that Ash, ever thoughtful, had spent weeks learning all about diamonds and their clarity and cut, and then had mine commissioned especially.

Everything was falling into place. All we needed now was a baby! Poor Ash, my perfect wishlist just never stopped!

Ash and I had always talked about kids but, up until a few years earlier, it had always been a case of 'in the future', or 'one day', a bit like the proposal.

For years I flirted with the idea of having children but, for a long time, I wasn't overly broody. Now I have a baby, I'm the complete opposite. I'd happily look after babies all day long as I understand them now. But, before, I think I had a lot of fear, which is silly really as, for lots of women, having children's such a natural thing to want to do.

Things started to change when I turned about twenty-eight. I began to crave a home life, marriage and babies. I think it's quite natural when it's happening to lots of your friends around you. When Ash and I got back together, we'd have long discussions about baby names and how we would bring a child up in the world.

But it wasn't until 2004, and I was thirty-one, that we started to talk about it quite seriously. To tell the truth, I'd been thinking about it for a while and, now that I was in my thirties, I didn't want to wait much longer.

When I mentioned it to Ash, he was really enthusiastic. 'Well, if that's how you feel, Becks, we should go for it,' he agreed. So that was that.

But then I got a call from my agent that changed everything. I had an audition for a part in *Casualty*. He sent over the script and, as soon as I read it through, I knew it was the part for me. Nina Farr was thirty-two, feisty, front-footed and passionate about her job. We sounded like evil twins! I told myself that I was going to get that part, whatever it took. I knew it was me. This was my chance for a real break – a move into mainstream TV on a Saturday-night show that pulled in ten million viewers – so I set about perfecting my audition preparation. Most actors and actresses sight-read when getting ready for a casting, but there were no second chances to impress with this, so I decided to take a risk and do my audition off the page (i.e. with no script, props or back-up). I had two days to prepare and, during that time, I did nothing else. The morning of the audition arrived. Ash made me breakfast, kissed me goodbye, wishing me luck, and I hopped on the train. Once I'd got to London and was on the tube, I decided to get into character as moody toughie Nina. No one dared shove me down the carriage or tread on my feet, that's for sure!

I arrived at the BBC and was put in a holding room with five other actresses who all looked just like Nina was supposed to, but I *felt* like Nina. I was 'in the zone'. I didn't talk to anyone, I didn't want to give away my energy; Nina wouldn't, I reasoned with myself. I remembered the eleven hours I had spent the day before at home, filming myself saying my lines and then playing the tape back, looking out for any tiny mistakes, recording myself on my Dictaphone and listening over and over again. I went over it all in my head, and then went in, ready to win.

I left the audition knowing I couldn't have given it any more. Now, I just had to wait. Three days later, I'd just been to see Ash at the garage, and was in my car, when my mobile rang. It was my agent, and I pulled over to answer it.

'Great news, Rebekah!' he said. 'You've got the job on *Casualty*!'

Oh my God! I was so thrilled that I cried – all that hard work had been worth it. I'd got it!

As soon as I had hung up, I turned the car around and drove back to the garage. I found Ash mooching around amongst the cars.

'What are you doing back here?' he asked me, bemused, as I skipped round a Mondeo, with a huge grin on my face.

'I've got *Casualty*!' I yelled jubilantly.

'That's brilliant news, Beck!' Ash replied instantly, beaming back at me. He looked so proud.

Getting a TV role was a massive deal, but it meant long hours filming, and not on my doorstep either. *Casualty* was filmed in Bristol – 150 miles and a three-hour drive from my home in Tunbridge. It was clearly no time to have a baby. Although I was broody, I still had my ambition, and I wanted the timing to be right. We agreed to put off the baby-making for another year or two.

I loved *Casualty* and soon immersed myself in my new role.

Often, there were big, long waits while scenes were set up, and it meant a lot of hanging around chatting with other members of the cast and crew, all part of the excitement of being on a TV show. We got to know each other really well, I spent more time with them than I did Ash! It became everything and I gave it one hundred percent.

But making *Casualty* was hard work. It was long hours filming, and I missed Ash even though he came down as often as he could.

Often, I'd be so exhausted that I'd stay in Bristol for the weekend or drive an hour and a half to Mum's place in Devon rather than face the three-hour trek back home to Tunbridge Wells. Living out of a bag felt quite empty at times, and I know Ash found it hard to deal with such an interruption to our domestic bliss, although, as before, we soon found a rhythm.

However, as time passed, I realised that I liked being at home, where everything had a place. I wanted to spend time with Ash, not to be filming miles away, much as I loved playing Nina, or going back on tour or into the West End. Working on *Casualty* was an amazing job – I knew I was so lucky to get a break on a show I had watched every Saturday night before I joined. It was my first TV gig, and I know how privileged I was to have such an experience and to have made so many dear friends. But, I had also learnt my lesson – I knew I couldn't put my relationship with Ash under all that pressure. I'd nearly lost him once; I couldn't risk it again. There's only so long it can all survive when you are never in the same room together. Plus, now, I *really* wanted a baby!

So, after almost two and a half years playing Nina, I felt it was time to move on.

We celebrated being back together with a holiday at the villa owned by Ash's parents in Marbella and then returned home to set up our life there once more.

A few weeks later, I landed a part in a play, and it was during that time that an actress friend really got me thinking. One night she confided in me that she now couldn't have kids. 'I missed the boat,' she said sadly. 'It's my biggest regret.'

Suddenly, it occurred to me that I was now thirty-four,

and my biological clock was ticking. Looking at my friend, all eaten up with sorrow, I just thought to myself, Gosh, we really need to get on with this.

There seemed no better time to start. Having a baby just felt like the next step – a natural progression. I no longer wanted my life to be just about my job, I wanted a family. And I didn't want to be an 'old' mum or, even worse, brokenhearted and childless because I'd left it too late. So, as soon as the play finished in October, Ash and I got down to business.

I was worried it might be difficult to conceive, so I was prepared to try very hard. I didn't have fertility tests or anything, but I had given up booze five months earlier and been on a big health kick – eating really good, nutritious food and doing lots of exercise, all in the hope it would help me have a baby.

I kind of knew when I was ovulating and had seen something on GMTV that said that, if you have sex a few days beforehand, you are more likely to have a girl. The report said that male sperm swim faster but die off quicker as a consequence, but the female sperm (those that contain the X chromosome) are slower, so will last out until you ovulate and have a jolly old crack at it.

So we had a go at that!

At times, I think I was a little over-enthusiastic.

Once, after sex, I did that thing, like in the film *Maybe Baby*, where you lie on your back and stick your legs in the air. I'm not sure that Ash thought it was very dignified. He just looked confused and mildly disgusted, so that was the end of that!

But, after a while, we got there and, in May 2007, we conceived our little Gigi.

I'd love to tell you a romantic tale of how Ash swept me off for a romantic weekend away and we held each other in a tender embrace on a four-poster bed scattered with rose petals. In reality, Gigi was the result of a heated argument and then a passionate make-up fumble in the spare room. Still, it did the trick!

When I first realized my period was late, I was actually training to do a half marathon for Cancer Research. I'd got up that day, drunk my energy drink, headed to the gym and started sprinting on the treadmill. But, after forty minutes, I couldn't run any more. I'd been training for ages, and it confused me. Then I looked at myself properly in the mirror, and realized my boobs were bigger too.

A wave of excitement tingled through me. Could I be pregnant?

I raced home, picking up a cheap pregnancy test on the way but, to my disappointment, it came up negative. Trying not to feel disheartened, I quickly threw the packet away and made myself a cuppa.

Over the next few days, I continued training, but I was perplexed to find I still couldn't run very far. I just felt tired, and my period was now a week late.

'I don't get what's up with me,' I confided in my friend Sarah when we met up for a coffee.

'Could you be pregnant?' she asked me.

I shook my head, but then I started to wonder. All the symptoms did point to one thing. Perhaps the test had been wrong?

So, right away, I went to the chemist's and bought a more expensive test. When I got home, Ash was out at work and the house was silent. I went straight into the downstairs toilet and peed on the stick.

Then I waited.

When the time was up, I looked down, biting my lip apprehensively. I could hardly believe my eyes – positive!

Feeling light-headed, I sat on the floor, still clutching the test stick. I felt as if the whole room was spinning. I've never been so emotionally freaked out.

Really, I should have just rung Ash and told him to come home before setting up some clever little display with the test. But I didn't. Instead, I rang my mum, and screamed, 'Oh my God!' down the phone.

She's pretty used to me being a drama queen, so she replied calmly, 'What?'

'Oh my God, Mum, I can't say the words!' I gabbled.

'Tell me,' she said, sighing.

'I really can't tell you!' I stammered. 'I really can't say the words . . .'

'Say them!' she snapped, now sounding justifiably irritated.

'I'M PREGNANT!!' I yelled.

Mum was clearly very, very shocked. She'd assumed I was going to tell her about a tour or a show or a TV role, like I always did. We've got a great relationship, and she's always very proud of me. She never wanted me to have babies too early, as she wanted me to achieve my dreams. Now, the revelation that she was going to be a grandmother clearly thrilled her.

'That's great news!' she trilled. 'I bet Ash is delighted!'

'Um, actually I haven't told him yet,' I replied.

'What?' she exclaimed. 'Well, phone him now, Rebekah!'

So, next, I called Ash.

'Are you sitting down?' I giggled. 'You better get home quick.'

'Why?' answered Ash. 'I'm on my way to the gym.'

When I blurted out the news, there was an eerie silence.

'Ash?'

'Right,' he finally spluttered. 'I'm coming home.'

Then, half an hour later, he burst through the door, grinning from ear to ear.

Both of us were delighted.

Being pregnant is weird. My body definitely felt different but, for weeks, I couldn't really get my head around the fact that there was a little baby growing inside me. Then, about ten weeks in, I began to notice a slight bump.

'It's our baby!' I smiled at Ash, placing his hand on my tummy. 'Can you believe it?!'

I had the usual morning sickness for a good couple of months, but it wasn't too bad at all. In fact, it was a time when I felt the happiest I'd been for years.

We were doing OK for money, so we made the decision to pay to have the baby delivered at the renowned Portland Hospital in London. The only problem was that it was an hour and a half trek from Tunbridge Wells into central London for each appointment. Consequently, when Ash and I went to hospital for my twelve-week scan, we had the biggest row over how long it took to get there.

Ash was agitated, as the scan came in the middle of a very stressful day at work, and I was annoyed with him for being irritable and not putting me and our baby first. By the time we got to the hospital I was doing my best to ignore him.

The twelve-week scan is obviously a very important one, so the pair of us were also on edge about that. We'd decided to go for the full monty and have all the blood tests which can highlight any abnormalities.

As we sat there, both tense and huffily ignoring each other, a girl came out of the doctor's office crying her eyes out. It was clear she'd just received some bad news. She looked inconsolable. It suddenly hit me that we couldn't take anything for granted. Having a baby was such a lottery.

Like all mums-to-be, I was anxious that my baby would be healthy and well, so seeing this poor girl distraught freaked me out. I tried to think calm thoughts, but it was no good. The first twelve weeks were so important. What if something was wrong with our baby?

Suddenly, Ash's voice whispered out from behind his newspaper. 'Everyone is on their own journey here, Becks,' he said, obviously wanting to make amends. 'Even if it's bad news, we'll do this whatever. Do you understand me?'

He sounded so serious that it instantly alleviated my fears and made me want to giggle instead. It was another Rocky Balboa moment. Little did I know at the time, but this would be the first of nearly two years of 'waiting-room moments', where we would sit and dread bad news, never knowing what we would find out.

Within half an hour, we'd been called in, and it was time to see our baby for the first time.

Thankfully, as far as the consultant could tell from our tests, there were no abnormalities, although I continued to fear the worst throughout my pregnancy, as the doctor explained that the result of the test for Down's Syndrome gave a 1 in 940 chance the baby could have it. But, during the scan, I tried to concentrate on the little heartbeat and the baby shape on the screen.

It was a beautiful moment. Ash squeezed my hand, and we grinned excitedly at each other, our cross words from earlier now forgotten.

Throughout my pregnancy I had some of the fairly normal cravings and some slightly more bizarre ones. I loved fish, chips and peas – well that's sort of logical, given fish is good for you and peas are great for folic acid. I also loved milk, and was addicted to cheddar cheese and pickle sandwiches – lots of calcium, good for the bones, or so I told myself as I tucked into my third one in a row! But then there was my oddball craving; I just couldn't get enough of the cleaning product Cif. I was constantly on a cleaning frenzy, and every bit of woodwork was washed with Cif. Ash would come home to find the house spotless and me practically sniffing the floors.

For a lot of my pregnancy, my hormones were raging. I had migraines, there were tears; I was a right old weeping wreck. To make matters worse, we had builders working on the house, right up to the week I gave birth, which made me very stressed. I just wanted to nest, but there was all this noise and disruption, and I was so unpredictably up and down. One minute I'd be crying hysterically, the next I'd be happy again. Poor Ash certainly had his work cut out!

But, aside from my horrendous mood swings, I think I got off pretty lightly. I'd heard stories from friends who'd had awful pregnancies where they felt wretched the whole time, but it wasn't like that for me at all. In fact, hormones aside, I felt positively blooming. Lots of people told me pregnancy suited me, and I felt pretty healthy; my skin was glowing and my hair had never looked better. Because Ash is quite old-fashioned and proud, he was adamant that he would support us through my pregnancy, that I should focus all my energy on growing our baby. He certainly didn't think it would be a good idea for me to be travelling long distances and dancing around on stage in high heels. So I didn't have to work, which felt weird after all those years of chasing down jobs and being on the road, but I soon slipped into my new role. I ate healthily and exercised as much as was sensible so that, in the end, I wouldn't gain too much weight. But my real aim was to get my body in the best shape it could be, ready for the birth. And, I figured the fitter I was, the quicker I would bounce back and feel really healthy to look after the baby once it was born.

Every day, I went swimming or for a lovely walk. I had the energy, but I would also rest when I needed to. I did everything I could do. I had early nights and, most afternoons, I went for a little catnap.

Friends often ask me now if I ever suspected something was up with me, if I had any inkling at all that I had cancer. But, before I discovered the lump, it was the furthest thing from my mind.

Yes, there were times when I was extremely tired, but I think it's well known that being pregnant in your thirties is very different from being pregnant in your twenties. A friend of mine had her first baby when she was twenty-six, and she sailed through it. When she had another at thirty-two, she found it a lot harder. So, when I did feel tired, I assumed it was down to the pregnancy, as you would.

Although I felt fine, I often found myself thinking very carefully about the future. When you are about to give life to another human being, I think you become more aware of your own mortality.

I certainly spent hours, days and weeks getting everything in the house in order. It was an instinctive thing. Every room needed to be sorted. I knew that, once the baby was born, I wouldn't have time to shower, let alone sort through boxes and drawers, so I just did everything.

Bizarrely enough, it was at this time that I began to prepare memory boxes for my child. I knew it was a bit morbid, but I felt it was important to put things from my past – programmes from my shows, photos, trinkets, the pregnancy test showing the positive result and love letters Ash and I had written to each other – together in a safe place. That way, if anything happened to me in childbirth, then there would be something left. Ash thought I was insane – he'd laugh and say, 'Christ, Beck, women have babies every day – it's not the eighteen hundreds any more!' But I just needed to do it. Looking back, I wonder if it was all part of 'a plan', if I was being driven to tie up these loose ends while I had the emotional space, before my world started crashing down around me. It's certainly not the most normal thing to spend your pregnancy doing. But, at the time, all I knew was that the memory boxes would enable my baby to know who Mummy really was if – God forbid – I wasn't around.

I read all the stuff about pregnancy and babies religiously – our shelves were groaning with books on every single stage of the pregnancy itself, and then guides on the first six, nine and twelve months. Feeding, changing, colic – even recipes for when the baby was weaned – I left nothing to chance. I didn't have a sniff of booze, I avoided soft cheeses, I kept out of smoky environments and I was obsessively washing my vegetables, fruit and salad leaves just in case of toxoplasmosis, which you can catch by being in contact with cat's poo and can really harm your unborn baby.

I saw my midwife once a week and was getting everything checked whenever I could. In fact, I became a bit obsessive, to be honest – a typical first-time mum. I suppose I couldn't believe how easy it had been to fall pregnant and, now, how great I felt.

'I just want to give our little one everything,' I told Ash as we lay in bed, him stroking my expanding belly, 'the best possible chance in life.'

Then, seventeen weeks into the pregnancy, I went for a scan on my own. It was just a normal ultrasound but, during the appointment, the consultant asked me whether I wanted to know what the sex of the baby was.

'Please tell me!' I said.

'Do you really want to know?' he asked.

'Yeah!' I enthused.

Up to that point, Ash and I had been dying to know. Ash already had bets going at work, and the people at the garage were split down the middle. I knew I'd be happy with either a boy or a girl but, secretly, the thought of dressing up a little girl in cute pink outfits excited me a lot.

Ash, on the other hand, was hoping for a son. He was already certain we'd have a boy, as was his mum. We'd already come up with a name for a boy, Ashley Junior, or AJ for short.

But should I really find out the sex without Ash being there? I knew he wouldn't really mind. Or at least I hoped he wouldn't! He'd known when I went off that morning that this was the scanning stage where they could tell what we were having. Ash also knows me well enough to guess I wouldn't be able to contain myself!

'Tell me, tell me!' I begged the consultant.

'Well,' he said, then paused. 'It's a little girl.'

'Oh my God!' I cried, hand to my mouth.

When the consultant nipped out of the room for a moment, I rummaged in my bag for my mobile and quickly typed out a text message to Ash.

'Know what it is!' I put.

By the time I got out of hospital, I had eighteen missed calls.

'I'm not going to tell you!' I teased when I called him back. Then I blurted out, 'It's a girl!' He was every bit as excited as I was. Suddenly, it all seemed so real. A little girl!

I couldn't stop smiling on the way home, imagining what she'd look like. Would she have Ash's eyes? My nose? I couldn't wait to meet her.

Now that we knew the sex, we immediately started discussing names in earnest. AJ was now out of the question, and we spent ages shouting out random girl's names. None of them seemed quite right until, one day, Ash just blurted out the name Gigi, which was also the title of my favourite musical.

'I love it!' I cried in agreement, and the decision was made.

We decided that Gigi was quite an extravagant name, so we tried to think of something we could derive it from – something a bit more traditional. We eventually settled on Gisele, and that was that: the bump now had a name and was well on her way to becoming a proper little person. It was overwhelming – so exciting!

Whenever Ash and I were out shopping together, I couldn't see a baby or childwear shop without going in and drooling over clothes, dollies, dummies – you name it!

'Put the bootees down, Rebekah,' Ash would laugh. But I'd pout and say, 'But Gigi wants them!'

Ash and I loved to spend evenings in, just the two of us, talking about what kind of upbringing we wanted for our daughter.

My mum had worked a fair bit when I was little, but I could still recall the delight I felt at having her at home, or her coming to pick me up from school – and we both wanted Gigi to experience that too.

At the same time, we'd both grown up with a strong work ethic, and it was important that she had that too and learned that things wouldn't just be handed to her on a plate.

It's funny how becoming a parent yourself really makes you think about your own childhood. I'd been affected very strongly by my parents' divorce. I really felt that I would never do that. I just didn't want that for my child. I wanted her to always feel loved and utterly secure. Love comes first, then a good education.

We'd already picked out a really good school and, provided she didn't have two left feet like her dad, I had my sights on her going to the local Tunbridge Wells branch of the Italia Conti performing arts school too. Poor kid didn't have a chance of being a tomboy!

Thinking about Gigi made me think back to how selfless my mum was when I was a child, always encouraging me or finding the cash for my drama or dancing pursuits.

'I want to support Gigi with anything she excels in,' I told Ash, and he nodded in agreement. 'I just want her to be an all-round good human being.'

As we discussed the secure life we'd carve out for her, how we'd travel, show her the world, give her happy times and shower her with love and affection, the future seemed so bright and perfect. How could we have ever envisaged what was just around the corner? How could we have known that, just as we were experiencing our most special time as a couple, my cells were dividing and battling to try and fight the cancer that was unfurling inside me?

It was the 23rd December and I was seven and a half months pregnant when I first felt the lump.

As my due date loomed, everything felt just magical, it was all going so well. I was getting totally fussed over by my friends and family and, as well as working my way through my bookshelves, I'd made a good circle of pregnant friends after joining up with the NCT (National Childbirth Trust). They were all first-time mums like me and, together, we went through the nervous excitement of what was happening to us and our bodies. It was so nice to be in a group, all of us at the same stage and worrying about similar things. Your body feels as if it has been taken over during pregnancy, and there was part of me that wondered if I'd ever feel normal again. But, on the other hand, I felt quite sexy and fit after all the swimming and walking I was doing. One reason I'd never felt better was also due to the fact that I knew Ash was loving me being pregnant. He never stopped telling me how great I looked, and that helped on the odd day when I felt like a beached whale.

We were ridiculously excited about having Gigi and had prepared a beautiful cream nursery for her. We had a gorgeous cot hand made, all specially carved with little acorns all over it and a canopy over the top. I mean, bloody hell, we had everything: steam sterilizers, bottle heaters, nappies – you name it. Everything was good to go. I don't think I had ever felt so settled and happy – and everything was made all the better by the fact that Christmas is my favourite time of year.

The tree was up, and I was contentedly writing all our Christmas cards in front of *Who Wants to be a Millionaire* on telly when I first felt it.

I had my hand rested on top of my tummy and I was stroking it absentmindedly when my fingers ran over a little lump on my left side, just above the bump on the underside of my breast.

By this point in my pregnancy, there had been lots of kicking and feet poking out so, at first, I didn't worry. I just thought, Oh bless, it's a little foot. But then, as I went on running my fingers across the lump, my stomach lurched.

My fingers traced the area under my breast, and I poked and prodded, hoping that Gigi would get the hint and draw her foot back in so I could relax. But the more I pushed and poked, the more I realized this wasn't to do with the baby, it was very different from what I normally felt. It wasn't a little foot or hand. It was a lump – the size of a walnut.

F***! What is that? I thought. Utter fear kicked in straight away.

4. A Lump and a Bump

The exact moment I found the lump is one of those moments that will be etched in my memory for ever. Quite often, I replay the scene over in my head. I close my eyes, and I am right back there, in front of the TV, writing those Christmas cards and feeling petrified as I desperately run my finger over the area around my baby bump and under my breast, willing the lump to disappear. That crushing fear has stayed with me; it's with me every day. Every time I check my breasts now, I hold my breath, replaying that initial discovery in my head as I pray my fingertips won't find anything. From the moment I found that lump, on 23 December, I have felt like a time-bomb just waiting to go off.

I was seven and a half months pregnant, very hormonal and very scared. When you're expecting a baby, you're obsessed with your body and notice every little thing that changes. I spent much of the first half of my pregnancy feeling like Dame Doom, on high alert for any sign that it could all go wrong. There are a lot of moments like that when you're pregnant. Suddenly, your body is a vehicle for someone else, and there is all this new stuff going on. I didn't recognize my body as my own at times and, just like most first-time mothers-to-be, I'd been completely paranoid about anything that seemed even remotely out of the ordinary.

My first real fright had been at five months. I'd been enjoying a girly lunch at my friend's home when I went to the loo and noticed tiny spots of blood. Immediately, I feared the worst – that I was about to lose my baby. I ran to tell my friends Sue and Sam.

'It's OK, Becks, it's quite common,' Sue immediately reassured me. 'My sister had exactly the same thing when she was pregnant and everything was fine. You just need to call your midwife and tell her.'

I called the Portland straight away and explained what was happening.

'Are you in any pain?' the midwife asked.

'No,' I replied.

'Well, try not to worry too much,' she said. 'Just monitor it for twenty-four hours and, if it continues, we'll need to see you right away.'

But, to my relief, the spotting went away almost as quickly as it had arrived, and soon everything was back to normal.

When you're pregnant, you spend so much time worrying 'what's this?' and 'what's that?' There is such a lot of information out there, too. I think part of the problem was that I read so much, my brain was just overloaded. Whenever I had a worry, I'd have to tell myself not to panic, as I knew getting stressed wasn't good for the baby. So, after the initial shock of finding the lump that December night, I knew I had to try to stay calm.

I shouted for Ash, who was in the kitchen. I pulled my top up and guided his hand to where I'd felt the lump.

'What do you think it is?' I asked him.

'I don't know, babe, but I'm sure it's nothing to worry about,' he told me, recoiling slightly. 'But you should probably go to the doctor's anyway.'

'Blimey!' he exclaimed as I put his hand back on the lump. 'It's really hard, isn't it? Does it hurt? Have you looked up in one of your books to see if it's normal?'

Ash wasn't really that into swotting up on what my body was going through and reading about all the ins and outs of pregnancy. I didn't mind really – it was my body, after all – and he was doing his bit in other areas, especially by working such long hours. But I could see that even he thought this felt a bit weird.

I tried to put it from my mind, but I could see and feel the lump as I got undressed for bed that night. It just felt so hard and angry. I lay in bed next to Ash, really trying not to panic, but it was scaring me, it just felt so alien.

I recalled what my friend Stef Spellman from *Starlight Express* had once said to me, that if a lump *doesn't* hurt, then that's when you should worry. When I pressed hard on mine, or pinched it under the skin, there was no tenderness whatsoever.

The more I thought about it, the more I felt sick, so I stopped touching it altogether.

'Oh come on, it can't be breast cancer,' I told myself. 'You couldn't be that unlucky!' Besides, my poor body was in hormone hell growing my baby – I was bound to spot unusual lumps and bumps. But still, I was well aware that you shouldn't mess around where lumps in your breast are concerned and decided to get it checked out anyway – no harm in getting peace of mind, even if the doctor would probably think I was fussing unnecessarily.

The next morning it was on my mind as soon as I woke up, so I called the doctor first thing.

The receptionist put me on hold to check if there was a spare appointment, I was praying she'd get me in that day. This is really important, and I can't wait until Christmas is over, I thought to myself. Inside, I felt all knotted. I just wanted to know that I was OK.

'Rebekah?' the receptionist came back on the line. 'I can get you in at eleven this morning.'

'Great!' I replied. 'See you then.'

When I arrived at the surgery later that morning, the receptionist greeted me with a big smile. The surgery looked all lovely and festive, but I couldn't focus on anything but the lump.

'Hi, how's it going?' she asked, no doubt assuming that I was there for a pre-Christmas baby check-up.

'Great!' I lied, smiling back at her with fake enthusiasm. I sat in the waiting room, rubbing my bump protectively.

'Please let it be OK, please let it be nothing,' I kept saying to myself, until, at last, my name was called.

Taking a deep breath, I stood up and walked down the corridor to the consultation room.

'How are you?' asked my doctor, smiling as her eyes travelled down from my face to my bump. 'When are you due?'

She'd naturally assumed I was there to talk about my pregnancy, too.

'Fourth of February,' I replied, then hesitated.

'Lovely,' she said. 'So what can I do for you today?'

'Look,' I went on. 'I'll cut to the chase. I've got a lump. I discovered it last night and it's worrying me.'

As I explained, the doctor's expression grew serious, mirroring my own.

'Well, take off your top and lie on the bed, Rebekah,' she said. 'I'll have a look.'

After I'd managed to heave myself up, she asked me to raise one arm, then the other, and examined me thoroughly, including all round my back.

I tried to think calm thoughts but could feel my heart racing in my chest.

'You can get dressed now, Rebekah,' she said, turning to wash her hands.

Putting my bra and top on quickly, I watched her silently, waiting for her to speak.

'OK,' she finally said, smiling. 'This is a blocked duct. I'm not concerned. I'll prescribe you a course of antibiotics, and that should soon clear it up.'

'Thank you,' I gasped in relief. 'That is such a weight off my mind. I really thought the worst there. I mean, when you think of lumps in breasts, you think of cancer, don't you?'

My doctor smiled again, handing me a prescription.

'No thanks,' I said. 'I'm sure it's fine, but I don't really want to take any medication while I'm pregnant.'

'OK. Well, just keep a close eye on it,' my doctor agreed. 'And come back and see me if it doesn't clear up of its own accord.'

Looking back now, I'm not actually cross that my GP didn't pick up on it straight away. After all, it's not like she misdiagnosed me on purpose. It was her job to calm a heavily pregnant and hormonal woman with a changing body, and that's exactly what she did.

However, leaving the surgery, I wanted one more reassurance, so I dialled the number of my friend Simone, who has three children.

'Did you get lumpy boobs during your pregnancies?' I asked, filling her in.

'Have you been to the doctor's?' she asked.

'Yes,' I replied. 'I'm just leaving the surgery now. My GP said it was a blocked duct and that I should go back if it doesn't clear up.'

'Well, then you'll be fine!' she said. 'Don't worry. Lumps and bumps are normal, especially if you think about all the strain on your body. Plus, the doctor said it was nothing, so forget about it and enjoy your last baby-free Christmas by putting your feet up while you can!'

Relieved, I called Ash to tell him the good news.

It was Christmas Eve, I had a beautiful baby bump and not a worry in the world.

Now we could concentrate on having a lovely, relaxing Christmas.

That night, at a family party, sipping my alcohol-free mulled wine and singing along with all my favourite Christmas carols, I felt happy and contented. The lump would soon be gone and life was good once more.

The next morning, I woke up feeling ridiculously excited. Traditionally, I headed home to Devon to be with Mum for Christmas but, this year, I'd decided to stay in Tunbridge Wells. By now, my nesting instincts were kicking in and I'd become a real home bird. The last thing I fancied was a five-hour drive to Devon.

I love Christmas. As mad as it sounds, we have about five Christmas trees around the house. The one in the bedroom is my favourite – our engagement Christmas tree where

Ash hid my ring. It is white and was covered in fairylights, and we had loads of fabulous things under the tree.

I've always loved giving and receiving presents, but nothing could ever be as exciting as opening Ash's gifts for our baby. The bump and I had done very well! Ash had really treated us, with all the dream items I'd wanted for Gigi's arrival. I had a Gucci nappy bag, relaxing Clinique candles, beautiful clothes, more baby books and bottles.

'You're a very lucky young lady!' I told Gigi, stroking my tummy.

Later, as we headed out to meet Ash's family, I looked in the mirror. I felt really proud of my lovely big bump, which I was enjoying covering up from the cold with big jumpers, woollies and gorgeous winter kaftans. Now that I'd been given the all clear, I felt good, really happy and so excited about what was to come.

We met up with eleven members of Ash's family at the Hotel du Vin in Tunbridge Wells for Christmas lunch. It was a raucous affair with lots of goodies and presents.

Although it's a modern hotel, that Christmas it had a really traditional feel, with log fires, loads of holly and a great big tree. There were lots of families there, and we soon joined in with random carols and cracker-pulling. Ash's family didn't stop for air. His cousins and their kids were there, all messing about and, as Ash held my hand, I couldn't help but think that, this time next year, our own little girl would be crawling around, into everything and part of it all. I couldn't wait.

By early evening, I was exhausted from all the excitement and from standing up all day, so we decided to bid everyone goodbye, then Ash and I headed home to snuggle up in front of the TV. It was the perfect end to a fantastic Christmas Day. It was the first time ever in all the years we'd been together that we'd both been at home for two full weeks – most years we were either staying with family, or one of us was working, so we really made the most of it. Thinking back now, it was almost as if we were given a capsule of time so that we could reconnect before the baby and the drama of the cancer. It was such a peaceful break and one that really helped me and Ash to strengthen our bond with each other before all the distraction and horror of the next few months – although, at the start, I did think that we might kill each other, as we weren't used to spending that amount of time together!

When New Year's Eve arrived, Ash and I celebrated with our dear friends Charlotte and Kit. It was just the four of us, and we had a wonderful dinner followed by chocolate fondue with marshmallows and strawberries.

Just before midnight, we huddled round the log fire and switched over to the BBC to watch the countdown.

It was really lovely and intimate and, as Ash cuddled me and stroked my belly, I just felt so content. It was already as if we were a real little family, and it wouldn't be long before the missing part was finally here. Then, at midnight, we cheered and had a big kiss as fireworks cascaded across the sky over the Houses of Parliament.

'2008!' Ash smiled. 'This is our new beginning, sweetie. This is our year. I feel so lucky about everything, Becks.' At that moment, we were both feeling very optimistic and excited about the future.

Although I loved that last month and a half of my pregnancy, I was also in this weird state where I just felt sad and teary. By the New Year, two weeks had passed since my visit to the doctor, but the lump was still as prominent as ever, and there was no change the following week either. Why wasn't it beginning to go? Why wasn't it sore? Perhaps it was a sixth sense but, deep down, I think I just knew it wasn't right. And I hid from the truth.

To the outside world, I was doing a great job of getting through the last weeks of pregnancy, but I was actually doing my best to hide my fears from everyone, including Ash. My neighbour Victoria, who was fast becoming a great friend, knew I had been to the doctor with a lump and, one day, as we were chatting over a cup of tea, she just asked me outright: 'You still got that lump?' I did my best to change the subject and told her that the doctor had said it was fine but, to tell the truth, I almost felt annoyed that she had brought it up. I didn't want to think about it.

A few days later, I was brooding on the sofa when Ash

came home from work. I'd spent the afternoon washing baby clothes in preparation for the big day, and I'd come across the memory boxes I'd made up a few months ago. Now more than ever they seemed so necessary, and I suddenly became engulfed by fear and started rifling through them. It was a shock to find that my life could be summed up in three cardboard boxes of mementos. Was this really all I amounted to, I wondered, beginning to convince myself I hadn't included enough for my daughter to ever know me after I'd gone. How the hell could any box be an adequate substitute for a mother anyhow? What if the doctor was wrong and I did have cancer? What if I died? I sat there running through every scenario – Ash would cope, of course he would, he'd survive without me; but it would be the hardest thing in the world to raise our baby alone. Even with loads of help from family and friends, he would be broken. And then I thought about the baby I hadn't even met yet. Every daughter needs a mummy – what if she lost hers before we had any time together? I began weeping uncontrollably. All the fear and anxiety was hitting me, the fragility of life suddenly felt so real. I couldn't cope.

Ash came in and saw the state of me. 'Becks, what on earth is the matter? Are you OK? Is it the baby?'

I looked up at him and just blurted out, 'If I died, Ash, you would be all right, wouldn't you? I mean, you would pick a good woman to look after you and Gigi?'

Ash looked at me as if I was clinically insane. 'What on earth are you asking that for, Becks?' he said.

'Nothing, I mean nothing much. It's just that this lump is still here.' I looked at him pleadingly. 'Feel it.' I watched his face as he registered the lump. 'Why hasn't it gone away, or at least shrunk? What if it's cancer, Ash?'

Whenever I touched the lump, it totally freaked me out. I'd run my fingers over it in the shower and shudder, or I'd be lying down in bed and I'd feel it and snap my hand away. I didn't want to prod it and make it worse, but I couldn't help myself.

I had brushed away any thought that antibiotics might help – there was no way I was going to put anything in my body that could spread itself through the placenta and into Gigi's system. In hindsight, since I was diagnosed with breast cancer, I've discovered there are some types of chemo that can be given to pregnant women once they are past the three month mark. But it would have killed me even to do that so, in a strange way, I'm glad I got the birth over and done with before I found out for definite.

Ash gave me one of his 'looks', and I knew I had to do something. He made me promise to call the doctor the very next day and get it seen to. I began to wonder if I had lost the ability to see sense – after all, the doctor had quite categorically told me there was nothing to worry about, and that the lump should clear up on its own. She hadn't said how long it would take – perhaps I was just being impatient? The problem was, the fear had taken hold. It was all too much to cope with this late into the pregnancy.

The next day was my baby shower, and I was delighted to have the distraction. So much planning had gone into this pink extravaganza, and all my friends were so excited that I just tried to throw myself into it. I had thirty-five friends arrive at the Spa Hotel in Tunbridge Wells for afternoon tea, and it was the campest thing I've ever organized.

I'd allocated jobs to several friends, and we'd all really gone to town. We had all Gigi's scans enlarged and put up, and there were pink ribbons and balloons everywhere. I even had a gorgeous pink cake with the name Gigi on it! I'd only ever been to one baby shower, but I just decided to really go for it. I loved all my friends for actually coming and indulging my madness.

We played games like guessing the baby's weight and time of birth. (When we discussed this later, Ash's dad thought I could give birth in half an hour – bless him for having such faith in me that I could pop her out in thirty minutes.)

My friend Michelle filmed the whole thing, and I asked all my friends to talk to Gigi on camera. From day one, I wanted Gigi's life to be filmed and photographed. I wanted every single minute of every day put down on record for her. So all of my friends, aunties, friends from *Starlight, Fame, Rocky, Copacabana* – they're all talking to the camera, giving her words of advice for the future. I always wanted to be big on those memories, but those taped messages would turn out to be very poignant just a few months later.

I was beside myself with happiness but, underneath it all, I still had a nagging feeling about the lump, and it hit me from nowhere when I gave a speech to thank everyone for coming. Looking around the room at all the women I loved and adored (and my mate Chris, who'd decided to invite himself, despite the fact that it was girls only!), I started to cry.

Being pregnant and hormonal, with all my closest friends around me, combined with dark thoughts about the lump, had made me realize how on edge I was. A little voice in my head was saying, 'I love these girls, why can't I just tell them the truth? That I'm happy about my baby, but I've also got a lump, and I am so worried it's cancer.'

But, as I tearfully surveyed my friends, I saw that they were crying and laughing at the same time, in that happy, emotional way people do at weddings. They thought I was merely crying with joy – the same old emotional Rebekah they loved, who'd cry at an *X Factor* audition.

'If anything ever happens to me, please tell my little girl about today and about me,' I sobbed. 'You're so special to me, and you're going to be so special to her.'

It was so important for me to have that for Gigi. It just occurred to me that my friends know me in a completely different context from the way Ash does. I think every one of your close friends reflects you in some shape or form. By the end of the do, we were all laughing the same dirty laugh, reminiscing and telling old stories from our younger days – it was just the tonic I needed.

It's a weird old thing when you are focusing on a new life but there is this underlying darkness. I knew I should sort it out sooner rather than later, but there was a battle of wills going on in my mind about this lump. The thought of scanners and hospitals and needles and tests filled me with fear for my baby. If I could only hang on until she was safely here, then at least I would know for sure that she hadn't been harmed. I was so tired, and everything seemed to exhaust and upset me. I just couldn't deal with it. 'Only a few more weeks,' I told myself.

Throughout our relationship, every couple of weeks I'd declare to Ash that it was time for our 'board meeting', which is our little routine of sitting down to chat about whatever needs to be addressed.

We do it basically so we can voice any concerns we've got or talk about something that needs doing. Before I was pregnant, Ash would raise his eyebrows at this, because it usually meant me nagging him about something – he always came off worse. But, while I was pregnant, he always used to play the game with me and say, 'Yes, sweetheart, what is it?'

So, one morning, I brought up the lump and said that it was still worrying me.

'What shall we do about it?' I asked.

I could see he was disappointed that I hadn't already made an appointment to get it checked out. He had been working day and night to clear his workload before the birth and earn some extra cash – truth be told, we'd been like passing ships in the night lately and had hardly seen each other since our idyllic Christmas. I'd told him I would get it sorted, but then I didn't and I didn't and I didn't, and I knew he was mad with me.

Eventually, he just shouted, 'For Christ's sake, will you just get a doctor's appointment? What is wrong with you?'

I shouted back and told him to drop it. 'I just need to get the birth out the way,' I snapped. 'I can't think about anything else, Ash. She'll be here any day, and then I'll get seen to. I've worked so hard to stay healthy for her, I don't want any stress or upset now.' He could see I was serious and getting really upset, so he decided to let it go. After all, Gigi would be here within a fortnight, and he had no idea what it felt like to be at the end of a pregnancy – as I kept reminding him!

As the day I was due to be induced – we lived an hour and a half's drive away from the hospital, and there was no way I was going to take the chance of Gigi being born on the A21 or the M25! – drew nearer, the lump was still there, but I continued to push the thought of it to the back of my mind, as there was so much to be done. There were last-minute antenatal classes to attend (which Ash avoided like the plague!) and lots of decisions to be made to fill my time. I was dragging Ash shopping, and he hated every minute! I was buying nappies, and I had no idea which to choose, Pampers or Huggies? I needed to get bottles, and I didn't know whether to use Avent or Tommee Tippee. And I also remember thinking, Should I get some grapeseed oil in case she has colic?

Then I would be buying baby-gros and wondering whether I should get whites so I could boil them up and put them on a hot wash, or pink because I was going to have a girl.

These were the things I was thinking about. That was the stuff I wanted to focus on at that time, part and parcel of growing a life and being about to give birth.

All my girlfriends from the NCT group I'd joined were beginning to drop one by one.

Each time we met, there was news of another baby, and the rest of us would still be waiting, nervously, and hearing the latest horror story. One girl would go off the scene, only to reappear three weeks later with her bundle of joy and an enviable flat tummy.

The last time we met was 29 January, the day before I was due to go into the Portland.

I was just like, Oh my God, this time tomorrow I'll have my baby!

Everyone was worried about giving birth, but my main concern was my baby's coming-out-of-hospital outfit! I also wanted Ashley all blazered up in a nice shirt and jacket. I remembered seeing David Beckham talking outside the hospital looking all dapper and handsome after Victoria gave birth to Brooklyn, and I wanted Ash to look just as suave. I'd ironed his best shirts and picked out all the sweetest little outfits for Gigi. I just wanted us to look like the perfect model family. I even imagined Ash smoking a calibre cigar outside the hospital, all cool and collected.

The way we drove into town to the Portland that night, all preened and polished, with matching Louis Vuitton luggage, it was as if we were heading off to Heathrow to go on a five-star trip. Of course, now that I've been through it, I realize that all the preparation and planning in the world can't prepare you for the stark reality of giving birth for the very first time.

In less than twelve hours, a worn-out Ash would be rubbing my back, looking pale and terrified, while I yelled every obscenity under the sun like a wild-eyed, screaming banshee.

5. Thank Heaven for Little Girls

There's a song by Luther Vandross called 'Dance With My Father'. It's so mellow and it reminds me of my mood in the hours leading up to Gigi's birth. It was actually playing in the car on Magic FM as Ash drove me to the Portland, and I remember feeling so happy and relaxed. Don't get me wrong – I was bricking myself, and so glad that I had chosen to be induced; it was really important to me to have some kind of control over something that was so life-changing – but I just kept turning to Ash and saying, 'You're going to be a daddy and I'm going to a mummy! Can you believe it!'

So here we were, at eight o'clock on a rainy evening in January, four days before my due date, making our final trip as a couple before bringing our baby daughter into the world and becoming a family.

There was hardly a car on the M25. Ash looked gorgeous in a smart jacket I'd laid out for him, and I was there with my big old bump wearing a tracksuit and Ugg boots. I kept thinking, This is the biggest day of my life! But rather than having a last-minute freak-out that I wasn't ready to become a mother, I felt very at ease and peaceful. I think it helped that I felt totally comfortable with the hospital.

After having so many appointments and really getting to know the doctors and midwives at the Portland, I had complete trust in the team of experts there. I know that some of my friends thought it was a bit unnecessary, going to a pricy private clinic, but I needed peace of mind. During my Dame Doom moments throughout the pregnancy, I became obsessed with all the horror stories I'd read of women and babies dying due to medical blunders, infections and maternity wards being understaffed. I know that paying for something doesn't automatically make it better or safer but, for some reason, going to the Portland made me feel that everything would be OK and, after all the angst of finding the lump, that was just what I needed.

When we arrived, Ash and I were shown into a lovely bedroom and I immediately set about unpacking all my clothes and cosmetics before changing into my pyjamas and climbing into bed. Now I was full term, I was very uncomfortable. The skin round my bump felt really tight, and my stomach felt so heavy. Carrying a good extra half a stone of weight in your tummy is ridiculously tiring, and I was relieved to put my feet up after the long and uncomfortable car ride.

Once I was all settled, at about 9 p.m., it was time to get cracking!

I was given an internal gel to start things moving and

then a sleeping tablet. This was the one and only time during my entire pregnancy that I actually agreed to take medication. I knew I was far too excited to go to sleep of my own accord, and I couldn't bear the thought of going through labour feeling exhausted before I'd even started!

Once Ash – who was staying near by at his sister Amber's place – had tucked me up in bed, he went to put his coat on. 'Right, I'm going to leave you to get some rest, babe,' he said, kissing me on the forehead. 'I'll see you in the morning.'

I lay there in bed for a while, feeling like a little girl the night before Christmas, until the sleeping tablet began to work its magic and my eyelids grew heavy.

I'm not sure what time I drifted off but, the next morning, I woke up at six, feeling an uncomfortable pain in my abdomen. Ooh, I thought, so it feels like this, does it? It was like a period pain.

After a nurse agreed that I was indeed in the early stages of labour, I rang Ash on his mobile and told him, 'You need to come in! I'm getting contractions!'

I was excited, but I felt a little bit apprehensive, too, so I was relieved when, at 8.15 a.m., Ash bowled in, accompanied by Amber.

'Have you got your cigar?' I joked. 'We have lift-off!'

I'd said all along that my mum would be my birthing partner, and Ash and I had kind of agreed that he would wait outside. I didn't really want him down there watching the head come out. I was worried it might make him see me in a totally new light, maybe even make him fancy me less. Ironic now given he's seen me at my worst. I mean, it really is a ring-side seat down there, and I sometimes think that women are so caught up in the whole thing while it's happening that we have no idea how it looks to a bystander!

Of course, friends had told me that Ash would want to be there at the birth, holding my hand, but I'd been insistent, saying that I would be happy with my mum being there.

I think it's normal to be a bit anxious, to feel that everything about your relationship will change with the arrival of a baby. Somehow, I worried that Ash would never forget the horrors of the birth, that it might mark the beginning of him forgetting me as his partner and equal – never mind the fact that Ash is totally squeamish and so was more than happy with my plan!

But, like all the best-laid plans, it all went to pot.

'I don't want anyone to get there until the afternoon,' I'd been saying all week. 'Nothing will happen for hours.'

So many of my friends had had long labours – forty-eight hours even – that I'd just assumed it would take ages for my baby to be born. Consequently, I'd told Mum to come up from Devon on the day itself rather than the night before.

However, it soon became clear that things were going to happen much more rapidly than I'd accounted for.

At 8.30 a.m. I was taken to the labour suite and, half an hour later, my lovely French consultant came to see me. He had the most fabulous accent – it almost took my mind off the agony I was in! He explained that I was not yet at the final stage of labour, but that it was time to take what he called his 'special magic pill', which would further induce the baby.

Half an hour or so after that, my contractions were getting quicker and more intense, but Mum had only got as far as Reading on the train. As time raced on, it became obvious that she probably wasn't going to make it for the actual birth.

'Don't worry, babe, I'm with you all the way,' Ash told me. But it soon became very clear that he was going to need his sister to hold his hand as much as I was going to need him to hold mine!

Bless Amber for hanging around. That day happened to be her birthday. It must have seemed a very novel way to celebrate!

By ten that morning I was in the final stage of labour and writhing around in pain, and Mum still hadn't arrived.

Ash put Magic FM on the radio in an attempt to relax me, and I had a bath, but the contractions were coming very fast, and I was astounded by how aggressive they were. I was sick a couple of times because of the pain and couldn't stomach gas and air. It just made it worse.

Then the pain got so bad that, by eleven o'clock, I was begging for an epidural. They called the anaesthetist and, although she was there within minutes, she had to give me a very detailed point-by-point rundown of it all – and that was on top of the half an hour the injection takes to kick in! But, by law, you have to be told about all the things that can happen to you, where they can inject you, what can go wrong . . .

I was getting in a right state: 'It's fine, it's all good – I've read a million books about what can go wrong. Just give me the drugs. Please,' I begged. As the anaesthetist continued with her catalogue of possible outcomes, Amber came to my rescue. Sensing I was about to scream the place down because of pain and red tape, she told the poor anaesthetist in no uncertain terms: 'Yeah, yeah, she understands and she definitely wants it!'

She administered the epidural, and the pain began to subside. It took a while, but then the agony was seeping away, then gone completely, so that all I could feel was the pressure of the crown of my baby's head. I just needed to free it with a couple of last teeth-grinding pushes.

Well, I could cope with that – just about! I had my knees at my ears, Ash squeezing one hand and Amber the other, and I pushed for a good twenty minutes.

As my labour progressed, I pushed and pushed and PUSHED. Oh, so much pushing! At times I felt so weary that I couldn't even speak, at others I was ready to scream blue murder.

I was very grateful that I'd swum thirty lengths religiously every day up to my admission. I'd heard that the fitter you are, the better the labour, although I can't honestly imagine it being much worse!

'I can't do much more of this,' I gasped to Ash, as he stroked my sweat-sodden hair.

'Yes, you can, babe,' he instructed in his best Rocky pep-talk voice, with Amber providing back-up.

'Come on, Becks, we're doing this together,' Ash soothed, rubbing my back.

I stopped and gave him my best filthy look! I mean, where on earth had that come from? For someone who hadn't attended a single antenatal class with me, he was suddenly a bit of a pro at this birthing lark, and very vocal about what I needed to do. It's weird now, when I think back: it's almost as if he was meant to be at the birth, despite what I'd planned. He was so great, despite my foul language, and it set the standard for how focused he remained throughout my cancer treatment – always scooping me up, telling me I could do it, urging me on.

And then there's the fact that he saw his daughter being born. There's no doubt that seeing every second of your baby's entrance into the world intensifies the bond you have. I am so glad that circumstances gave him that – especially if anything happens to me. Sometimes I look at the two of them snuggled up together, and I know that it all happened for a reason, that he's a better father for having been there for her grand entrance. It's so important that we shared the same experience and that, if I'm not here to tell Gigi all about it, then he can.

'Keep breathing, Becks,' he instructed. I guess all those *Casualty* episodes I made him watch had their use after all. Suddenly, he was a regular Harry Harper!

'Where's Mum?' I panted.

'Don't worry about that!' Ash urged, rubbing my back and squeezing my hand. 'Just push, sweetheart!'

Another twenty exhausting minutes of flat-out pushing and then, with one last heave, the head was clear and she was there! My labour had been just under three hours long.

As I lay there, every part of me throbbing, gasping for breath, the midwife placed Gigi gently on my breast. Studying this tiny little person for the very first time, I held my breath. She looked so small and had this slightly stunned look on her face, yet she seemed very calm and content. She seemed wise, too, as if she were scanning the room, taking in everyone there.

I was speechless, and I looked up at Ash and Amber. They were both stood there gazing at her with wonder and so overcome that they were openly crying. Gently, I ran my fingers over her downy little head, completely amazed by her.

'Hello, Gigi,' I whispered.

The whole thing was overwhelming. As most besotted new mums will agree, I felt consumed by love straight away.

Later, writing in Gigi's baby book, I summed up her arrival with, 'You were warm, calm and loving.'

She was just perfect. My beautiful little girl.

For the next half an hour we had staff coming in and out to check on Gigi. They scratched her feet to check all her senses, weighed her and gave her her vitamin K injection.

Then, from 12.30 onwards, our parents started arriving.

Ash's dad, Rod, is a big, tough man, and he arrived in his shades and jacket, followed by Ash's mum, Jen.

'What's going on then?' he asked gruffly, surveying the paraphernalia of the room but, comically, not noticing little Gigi clamped to my breast. She'd latched on straight away and had a very healthy appetite. It was such a big moment, giving my baby her first feed, that it didn't occur to me I had my breast out in front of everyone! As soon as she had finished her feed and was dozing, a smiling Ash gently lifted his daughter out of my arms and presented her to his parents.

'This is Gigi,' he said.

There wasn't a dry eye in the room. Ash's parents circled him as he held his daughter, and Amber took loads of photos. It was so sweet to see Ash proudly showing off his little girl.

Then, just as everyone was beginning to compose themselves, we told Ash's sister that we were giving Gigi the middle name Amber, after her.

'That's the absolute best birthday present I've ever had,' she exclaimed. And then everyone cried again.

'What time was Gigi born?' Jen then asked.

'11.50 a.m.,' I replied.

Her face looked completely shocked.

'Are you sure?' she asked. 'That's exactly the same time Amber was born!'

It was so spooky, and I don't think I really believed them until days later, when Amber showed me her birth card. But there it was in black and white. There's always going to be a special bond between those two, I think.

Then, a little bit after that revelation, Mum finally arrived.

'Oh my God, you could have waited for me!' she said, laughing as she rushed in with all her baggage.

She looked like an excited little girl and, for me, it was just the cherry on the cake to see her. When she came over to kiss me I could smell her perfume, and it was really comforting.

'Oh, she's beautiful!' she exclaimed. 'She looks the spit of you as a newborn!'

'That's funny, because Jen's convinced she looks just like Ash,' I laughed.

But Mum didn't mind. You couldn't wipe that smile off her face.

As everyone drank tea and had toast with marmalade, Mum recounted how she'd jumped in a taxi at Paddington and said, 'Put your foot down, please, my granddaughter is being born!' She loves a drama. It must run in the family!

I just lay there listening to everyone chatting away – this mêlée of noise and happiness. I still felt a bit dazed from the epidural, and all those feeling-good, healing hormones were kicking in too.

We were on a floor really high up at the Portland, and the sun was gleaming in through the windows. The radio was still on, and there were lovely soul tracks playing. It was amazing. My only wish was that my dad could have been there, too, but we'd agreed he would come up later. I wanted it all to be calm around my precious girl, and there was plenty of time for the two of them to meet.

After a while, my midwife wanted me to get cleaned up, so she shooshed everyone away for lunch. She ran me a bath, swaddled Gigi in a little white sheet and put her down to sleep peacefully in her cot, then she left me on my own to have a bath.

With the room quiet and all the banter gone, I lay there with the most satisfied glow. I wasn't thinking about anything. I just wanted to wallow in happiness.

Then Gigi started crying. Well, that was the first time I'd ever heard her cry – and talk about maternal instinct! It was like I'd been zapped with a laser gun! I shot out of that bath, grabbing a towel, and limped, damp-footed, across the room to her cot.

I picked her up, so scared at how tiny and vulnerable she

was, and sat on the rocking chair next to her cot. As I sat there soothing her and getting to know her, the sun was still blazing through the window. A beautiful song called 'Heaven', by Bryan Adams, came on the radio, and Gigi immediately stopped crying. It was magical. It was as if the lyrics summed up all my emotions and all my love for my little baby. I just sat there looking down at her, crying.

It really did feel like heaven to be holding her, and I decided from that moment that it would be Gigi's special song. It's also a song that would give me a certain amount of comfort during my treatment. When I felt dreadful and things were tough, I used to put it on the stereo, and it would remind me that I didn't want my little girl to grow up without a mummy there for all those big and special moments. Whenever I felt worn down by it all, it reminded me I had to fight.

Over the next couple of days, the amazing staff at the Portland took so much care in easing me into motherhood. It was far less daunting than I'd imagined it would be. The nurses were all maternal types, aged between forty and sixty, and it was like having a team of professional mothers looking after you.

There was this one lovely night nurse called Jackie who was brilliant at helping me through those first few 3 a.m. feeds.

'Gigi, come, come,' she'd say softly, rubbing my baby's little cheeks to wake her up when she drifted off during a night feed. I still say, 'Come, come,' to Gigi now.

While we were in the hospital, lots of friends came to visit, and they showered us with flowers, chocolate and gifts. My phone rang constantly.

My favourite thing was going into the nursery and catching up with all the other excited mums who'd just given birth.

When Gigi was a day old, Ash and I were given a lesson in how to bathe her by a strict Scottish midwife.

Ash was taking it very seriously, asking all the really sensible, proper questions – Which babywash do you use? How do we test the water? What are the different ways you can hold her? – while I was too busy squealing, 'Bless her, having her first bath!' and taking photos of it all, Ash shooting me warning looks.

On our last night at the Portland, I put Gigi in the nursery so I could get some rest but, at 5 a.m., I woke up, hearing the hustle and bustle of the London traffic below. Except, that wasn't what had woken me. I was sure I could hear Gigi crying, but that was impossible, as the nursery was right down the other end of the corridor. Still, it unnerved me and, within minutes, I'd jumped out of bed and was racing down the corridor in my T-shirt and pants.

Sure enough, when I burst into the nursery, I saw that she was crying (to be fair, so were about three other babies) and I ran to pick her up to soothe her.

The thought that she'd been crying for me in the nursery was awful, and I vowed then and there that I'd never leave her again while she was so small and vulnerable, unless it was a matter of life or death. And what a poignant promise that turned out to be!

I found it a real struggle to leave the Portland the following morning.

I always like to give Ash the impression that I can cope with anything but, on the third day after giving birth, your hormones are crashing, and the happy, euphoric feeling is beginning to drift away, as the reality of the mammoth task in front of you begins to sink in. Plus, now the birth was over and I had started breastfeeding, I knew I could still feel the lump in my breast, and that I would have to speak up and deal with it. However, it really isn't a cliché to say that you don't get a minute to yourself once you've had a baby – it's all you can do to mastermind going for a pee. We were just in this gorgeous bubble – me, Ash and our Gigi. It felt ridiculous to think that anything could ruin it for us.

Our room was scattered with so much stuff – cards, flowers, gifts and all the baby bits and pieces we had already accumulated – but, as I tried fruitlessly to create some sort of order to my belongings, Gigi kept crying, and I felt totally overwhelmed by everything. Luckily, one of the lovely midwives came in and instantly calmed us both down. I was scared shitless when it was time to leave, but I also knew I had to learn to look after Gigi without all that extra help.

All too soon it was time for Ash to pick us up from hospital to take us home. Together, we tucked Gigi into her car seat. She was wearing the little outfit I'd chosen especially – a cute white baby-gro with matching bonnet – and I covered her in a thick white blanket to keep her warm in the bitter February chill.

I sat in the back with her, and she slept for two hours solid, all the way home. We didn't hear one little murmur. She just looked so tiny and adorable in that car seat, like a little doll, and I couldn't take my eyes off her.

We arrived home at 2 p.m. and carefully carried Gigi into the house. It was so surreal finally to have our little angel at home. We'd been preparing for months and, now, here she was, and she was perfect. Gigi and me cosied up on the sofa, and Ash went out to get provisions. We wanted to settle in for a long weekend, but knew we'd have lots of visitors, so we stocked up on goodies and cakes.

For ages, I didn't put Gigi down but then, when she grew sleepy, I swaddled her and put her in her Moses basket.

'Ash, look at her!' I whispered.

'Do you think she'll actually be able to grow if you swaddle her that tight?' he whispered back, grinning. 'You haven't cut off her blood supply, have you?!'

That night, as I gazed at her sleeping, I couldn't stop smiling to myself.

★ ★ ★

That first blissful day at home was such a beautiful time.

Ash and I were completely besotted with Gigi, and it really felt like nothing else mattered. From the day our daughter was born, our whole perspective on life changed.

I'd worried about all sorts of things in the past. I'd been concerned about what people thought of me, or my career, or loads of other silly little things but, from the moment Gigi came into the world, that all stopped. But, as I began to get used to life as a new mum, there was one nagging worry still there – the lump in my boob.

From the moment I'd nursed Gigi on the first night, I knew that blocked duct was still there – I could feel it – and, over the next couple of days, it didn't disappear. In fact, I was sure it was bigger now, and it still didn't feel tender when I ran my fingers over it.

One night in that first week, as I was feeding, Ash came in and caught me examining it for the millionth time. He frowned at me with concern and a bit of irritation.

'Rebekah, you must go to the doctor's,' he told me, trying to keep his voice down so as not to disturb Gigi. 'Please make another appointment. If you don't, I will. I've had enough of this – it's mad. Just go, will you? I know they said it's nothing, but get peace of mind and let's move on. You said you wanted to wait until Gigi was born before you went to get checked out again. She's here now – what's stopping you?'

So I called the doctor's and arranged to go the following

day. Because Ash was back at work, I made a loose arrangement for Ash's mum to come over and take us in but, fifteen minutes before the appointment, Jen still hadn't arrived, and I couldn't get in contact with her.

I suppose I could have just put the baby in the car and driven there myself but, at that stage, I was still finding my feet, and everything about motherhood seemed very daunting. I was anxious, weepy and unable to cope with it all.

When people meet me, they often think I'm really confident but, like everyone, I have moments of self-doubt and timidity. It sounds silly but, at that point, what with getting used to looking after a baby, I couldn't build up the confidence to leave the house. I found the whole experience completely overwhelming.

The idea of attempting to get Gigi out of the house and loading her into the car, with everything she needed – well, it was as if I had to have a degree or something. I was still in pain, and had previously had no idea that I would bleed so much and for so long after giving birth. Plus, I'd hardly slept a wink since coming home, and I felt so weak and tired. I was just a bit numb with it all.

I'd even had a moment in the shower that morning when I'd lost my balance and nearly fallen. I was a bundle of nerves. But I knew how important the appointment was so, when I missed it, I just sat there and sobbed.

I'd been told that, in the weeks after the birth, I could experience erratic mood swings and, at that moment, it honestly felt like I was trying to fight the world. I was attempting to stay happy, but I felt completely overcome by the practicalities of having such a tiny thing depending on me for everything.

By the time Jen did arrive, after being held up in traffic, a huge sense of dismay had swept over me. Looking back, it was nothing but a pretty minor case of the baby blues, but I felt totally incompetent and crap. And I also knew Ash would be on my case about getting another appointment so, taking a deep breath, I called up the surgery and asked them to reschedule.

They gave me an appointment for 21 February – over two weeks away. When Ash got home, he could see the state I was in and how exhausted I was, and that, combined with the fact I had booked another appointment, meant he wasn't too mad with me. After all, he'd only got angry out of concern for me.

Up until the time of the next appointment, I put the lump to the back of my mind once more. I just got on with trying to break through the breastfeeding pain barrier and learning to express my milk. The whole process of feeding and expressing brought me out in a cold sweat, but I really wanted to do it, as all the books say it is best for the baby. My breasts were extremely tender at first (bless Ash's cousin, who bought me a Savoy cabbage, telling me to put it in the fridge, peel off the leaves and put them in my bra. It's really soothing on your boobs; it worked a treat and brought me some much-needed relief), but Gigi latched on and was feeding very well, even from the boob with the blocked duct.

I'm sure some women are pretty relaxed with breast-feeding, but I had very little confidence that I'd ever get to the stage where I could just sit in a restaurant and flop out a boob. They'd ballooned to a 36FF, for goodness' sake! I certainly didn't want to get those pendulous monstrosities out in public! I felt very self-conscious about the whole thing so, if I needed to go out or do a shop, I used to express off. I found it easier that way.

I would like to say I was this confident thirtysomething mum, completely in control, but I wasn't. Now that I think about it, although I bounced back physically, emotionally I really struggled. Thank goodness I had such a great support network around me.

Jen would come over and whack the hoover around, or get some shopping in. I craved crab sandwiches – I hadn't allowed myself to eat shellfish while I was pregnant – and so she'd make a special effort to get them for me. She was an angel.

Mum had headed home the day after Gigi was born but came back up soon after and stayed for a week. It was she who gave me the confidence to get dressed and head out the door. I'd feed Gigi first, then we'd go for lovely walks in the fresh air, and then for tea and cake.

Then, when Ash's mum went to Spain and my mum

went back to Devon, it was my lovely neighbour Victoria who stepped up.

Having all these amazing ladies around really helped. When you don't know what you're doing as a new mum, it's other women's advice you need, and Mum, Jen and Victoria really were my lifeline.

Three weeks after Gigi's birth, Jen had Gigi for me, and I FINALLY made it to the doctor's surgery. This time, I saw a locum doctor, which I was pleased about. Now I could get a second opinion without my own doctor thinking I was neurotic, and perhaps it would put my mind to rest once and for all.

Mirroring my previous appointment, the locum doctor examined me (which now wasn't easy, seeing as my breasts had doubled in size!). She didn't seem concerned at all and was really friendly, chatting away about Gigi and breast-feeding as she took a good look at everything. Afterwards, she seemed satisfied, and told me: 'Pregnancy does strange things to your body. I think it probably is a blocked milk duct.'

At first, relief washed over me. After three weeks of interrupted sleep, 99 per cent of me really wanted to accept what she said, to take this comforting verdict and get back to my newborn baby. But there, niggling away at the back of my mind, was still that 1 per cent doubt. Despite rationalizing that I had now had two professional all clears from two separate doctors, my gut instinct was telling me to be wary.

'I'd like to get a referral,' I told her. 'Just for peace of mind.'

The locum didn't seem to mind that I was asking for a second opinion and, once she'd agreed to set the wheels in motion, I also asked her if she could recommend a private consultant. I explained to her I wanted to get seen as soon as possible, so that I could stop worrying about it for good. She gave me the number of a doctor at the local hospital.

When I left the surgery, I felt all fired up and called the consultant's office straight away and explained my situation.

His secretary was less than helpful.

'I'm sorry. We see people a little further down the line,' she told me, a bit flippantly. 'Why don't you wait for your referral?'

'Oh, OK,' I said, deflated.

Looking back now, I don't know why I took no for an answer. Two months had passed since I'd noticed the lump, and I was still none the wiser about it really. Alarm bells were ringing in my head, but I let that woman knock me back just like that. But, at that point, I really felt as if I was going crazy, banging my head against a brick wall. I was exhausted, totally worn out, and I didn't have the energy to make a big fuss.

It might not have been big or clever but, once I did finally get diagnosed with breast cancer, I actually called that woman back and tore shreds off her.

I recognized her voice as soon as she answered, but I could tell she had no idea who I was.

'Hi, my name is Rebekah Gibbs. I called a couple of weeks ago about a referral.'

There was a pause, as if she was going through her memory to try and pull out my name from the back of her mind.

'Hmmm, Rebekah Gibbs, Rebekah Gibbs,' she said, as if repeating my name would help her remember.

'You told me,' I interrupted, 'that you didn't see people until they were "further down the line".' I paused. 'So, explain to me, at what part of the line does it become important to see a woman with a lump in her breast, especially when that woman is offering to pay?'

I'm sure she could tell right away from my tone that something was wrong. 'You were quite flippant, actually.'

I knew I was being sarcastic, and a bit unfair, I knew she wasn't to blame for what was happening to me, but I couldn't help it.

'Oh yes, I do remember you.' She seemed uncertain and wary about where this conversation was going.

'Well, I have just been diagnosed with cancer. I hope you're happy!' I screamed. 'You refused me an appointment when I had grade-three cancer!'

There was a shocked silence.

'I – I—' She was stumbling over her words, but I didn't give her the chance to collect herself; it was as if I was possessed.

'Do you realize what you have done to me?'

Well, that time, she'd bothered to listen, and then she apologized profusely. She sounded upset; she was just a woman like you and me – it wasn't her fault. But when I'd finally slammed down the phone and slumped on to the sofa, I felt a sense of relief. It may have been futile but, at my worst moment, I needed to let my frustrations out and, unfortunately for her, she was an easy target.

If I thought I could just go home and forget about the lump after that first conversation with the consultant's secretary, though, then someone up there was trying their damn hardest to spur me into taking action. Just after I'd been to see the locum doctor, a friend of mine told me a shocking story over the phone. She was upset, as a pal of hers had died, and – yes, you've guessed it – it was breast cancer that had killed her.

'She found a lump in her breast, but her GP turned her away,' my friend revealed. 'Within a year, she was dead. Can you believe that?' I tried not to cry as the conversation ended but, when I got off the phone, I instantly burst into tears and went to tell Ash. I felt utterly crushed. I suddenly realized that, in a year, someone could be talking about me in the same context. That could be my fate, too.

Wanting to protect me, Ash's initial reaction was anger that someone would relay a story like that to me when I'd just had a baby and was so emotional and hormonal.

When I'd wiped my eyes, I leapt to her defence.

'She didn't know about the lump,' I sniffed. 'It's probably a good thing she told me, she wasn't being malicious.'

Ash stared at me as if he had known exactly what I was going to say.

'I needed a short, sharp, shock like that,' I added, blowing my nose. 'It'll make me go to the doctor's again.'

'Well, make sure you do,' he said softly. 'I'll come with you for back-up. It might help?' And we agreed that that's what we would do.

A few days later, before I had done anything, my hospital referral came through for 7 April. I considered trying to get another appointment before that, but what could I do, really? Two doctors had told me it was nothing, I'd been knocked back by the local private hospital and now I had a referral. Should I make a fuss simply because I had a funny feeling it was something more sinister than a blocked milk duct?

'You obviously can't beat the system,' I told myself. 'That's the appointment I've got, so I'll just have to wait.' In a sense, I think I felt like I couldn't really kick up too much dust, as I'd waited a while before going back at all. To be honest, I felt a bit silly.

Before I knew it, three weeks had flown by, in a blur of

baby sick, dirty nappies and sleep deprivation, and now it was 14 March, the day we were off on a much-needed break to Ash's parents' holiday home in Marbella. And, in those weeks, I didn't have any time to worry about my own health anyway, as Gigi was worrying me immensely. She had terrible colic. It was proving to be quite a testing time.

In fact, just days before we left, I was actually considering cancelling our trip, as she was really suffering. She'd cry for two hours almost non-stop and would go really red in the face. It was terrifying, and very upsetting to watch – I hated seeing my baby in so much pain when I couldn't do anything to help. It would get to 9 p.m., and neither of us would have eaten all evening, because she was so bad. It was a different cry from her usual one; it sounded really strained and painful, and nothing seemed to soothe her. I kept saying to Ash, 'I don't know what I'm doing wrong. What do I do?'

Thank goodness, though, she did settle down a little, just before we left.

Marbella was going to be Gigi's first holiday, and we were also celebrating my thirty-fifth birthday while we were out there. As an early birthday treat, and to make our first flight with a colicky baby easier, Ash paid for us to fly out first class, for a bit of luxury, and I was determined to enjoy myself. Once again, not knowing how else to cope, I pushed all thoughts of the lump to the back of my mind. It was the only way I could make the most of my holiday. Anyway, I had my appointment in the diary, and I couldn't do any more before that.

Once we were there, Ash's parents were only too eager to help with Gigi, which was such a relief. The colic had been exhausting and had really made me doubt my ability to cope, so it was good to have a safe pair of hands like Jen's helping through the whole process. She and Rod were amazing, always asking if they could take care of Gigi, so we were able to get lots of rest and sunshine and really catch up on our sleep.

On my birthday, we went to Orange Square for paella, taking Gigi with us. It was beautiful out in Marbella in March, and we watched the sun go down in complete peace and harmony.

By the time our ten-day break was almost up, amazingly, any thought of the lump had evaporated from my mind. I felt totally chilled. We both did. We'd really recharged our batteries, and it had been fantastic relaxing in the sunshine with our gorgeous little girl. The luxury of sleep had given me back some spark and, by the end of the holiday, I was even breastfeeding in restaurants. I felt utterly blessed. But then, just as we were about to come home, everything changed.

We were taking Gigi for a little stroll around the villa's garden when Ash received a phone call from Richard, a good friend of ours from back in Tunbridge Wells.

I could tell immediately by the tone of Ash's voice that something bad had happened.

'I can't believe it,' I heard him say. 'How's Madeleine taken it?' Madeleine was Richard's wife.

Putting the phone down, Ash looked pale. 'Madeleine has just been diagnosed with breast cancer,' he said.

'Oh my God, poor Madeleine,' I replied, covering my mouth with my hand.

It beggared belief. She was only thirty-six, and she had two little boys. How could this be happening to her? Then fear shot through me as I remembered my own circumstances. I felt completely winded.

Walking over, Ash put his arm round me and Gigi, and we had a little group hug, just the three of us. He didn't say anything; he didn't need to. He just looked at me, with sadness in his eyes. As well as being upset for Madeleine and Richard, I knew the same fear was racing through him as it was me. There was no escaping the fact that I had a lump just like Madeleine had. The doctors had told me it was fine, but it was still really worrying me, and I still hadn't been checked out properly.

My hospital referral was two weeks away, but I needed an answer now. Why was I allowing this to go on for so long? I needed to be proactive but, when you're scared, there're always a trillion things to do first, aren't there?

By the time we got back to England, Madeleine had already had her lumpectomy. A few days had passed, and I still hadn't called the doctors. I didn't want to go back to my GP, in case I was facing the same diagnosis as Madeleine, so I stalled – cleaning the house, catching up on paperwork – basically anything to put off the inevitable.

The weekend was now looming, and I'd done nothing. And it was after Ash had been to see Richard for a drink on the Friday afternoon that he finally really flipped out on me.

Ash never really shouts but, when he walked in the door and discovered I still hadn't made an appointment, he was fuming.

'Will you please just sort it out!' he told me, his voice getting louder with frustration. 'What are you waiting for, Becks? What on earth are you waiting for? In fact, don't bother to even speak to me tomorrow if you haven't made an appointment. Enough is enough. There's so much at stake. Just look at what's happening with Madeleine.'

At this point, more than three months had passed since I'd first spotted the lump and, although I'd been reassured it wasn't anything to worry about, I knew I couldn't delay any longer. So, the following Monday, 31 March, I went back to see my doctor, the GP who'd first given me the all clear. My hospital referral was in a week's time, so I figured I'd talk about Gigi first, then mention the lump.

Arriving at the surgery early, I parked and looked up Madeleine's mobile number. She and Richard had flown off to Tenerife to help her recover from her surgery, and I knew the last thing she would want to do would be to talk about lumps and breast cancer, but I couldn't think what else to do. I was desperate to speak to someone who knew what I was going through. It took me three attempts before I could bring myself to press dial. I felt sick with nerves.

'Madeleine, I hope you're OK and I'm so sorry to bother you while you're away,' I apologized. 'And I know it's probably not what you want to hear, but I've got a lump too.'

'Oh, God, Rebekah. How long have you had it?' she replied.

'Um, about three months,' I admitted. 'Two doctors have said it's fine, but I wanted to ask you what yours felt like.'

As Madeleine began to describe how she'd found her tumour in the side of her left breast, under her armpit, I began to tremble. Then she told me how it didn't hurt at all, especially when she touched it.

I felt nauseous. It sounded exactly the same as my lump.

'Rebekah,' she instructed me. 'I'm going to text you the name and number of my consultant. Now, promise me you'll get it sorted. Please promise me.'

When I was off the phone, I took a deep breath. Things seemed bleak, but a little part of me was still trying to hold on to the thought that two doctors had looked me in the eye and said the lump was nothing to worry about.

As I walked into the surgery, carrying Gigi in her car seat, I heard my phone bleep with Madeleine's text. Sitting down, I grabbed my mobile out of my bag and switched it off. Then I sat there, telling myself, 'It'll be OK. She'll tell me it's nothing.'

When my name was called out I walked into the doctor's room, and she greeted me with a warm smile. 'How old is she now?' she said, indicating Gigi.

'Nearly ten weeks,' I replied. But then I changed the subject. 'I wanted to ask about that lump you looked at while I was pregnant,' I said. 'You see, it's still there, and I wondered if you could take another look, just for my peace of mind? I really don't feel happy about it.'

'Let me see,' she answered, frowning slightly.

Once again, I took off my top and clambered up on the couch. We went through the same procedure as before, with her examining the lump thoroughly.

I think I'm intuitive, I can often read people's faces and, in the doctor's, there was definitely something I didn't like. I could tell instantly that I wasn't in for good news. Straight away, her face froze. Her hands went back and forth over the lump and the surrounding area. She told me to get dressed and, while I did, without saying a word to me, she got on the phone. I could hear the dial tone. She looked a bit panicked. I felt sick to the stomach. This was bad, bad news.

She looked up and met my eye briefly. 'I'm going to see if I can get you to the local hospital today,' she said. 'I'm concerned.'

I looked at Gigi, sitting, oblivious, in her chair, then cleared my throat. 'Hold on a minute,' I said. 'Has it changed a lot since the first time I came? Is it bigger? Why are you worried now when you weren't then?'

She continued to wait for someone to pick up the phone at the other end.

'If the lump had felt like this in December, would you have referred me straight away?' When she answered, 'Yes,' I couldn't wait to get out of there.

The doctor had a hurried conversation on the phone, while I got more and more impatient and scared. The atmosphere in the room became very grave very quickly.

'I can't get you in today, but I can tomorrow,' she said, once she'd hung up. 'I'll sort it out for this week, and I'll be in touch with you.'

'No,' I replied, feeling my eyes begin to well. 'I'm getting it sorted today.'

Ash's words were ringing in my ears, and I knew that this was serious. I didn't need the doctor to say anything else to know I was in trouble.

Then I walked out and sat in the hallway of the surgery, crying my eyes out.

Almost immediately, poor Gigi started bawling too, so I tried my hardest to calm her while I fumbled in my bag for my mobile. Finding it, I quickly scrolled to Madeleine's text message and found the number for her consultant, Mr Williams.

'Please help me,' I sobbed, when his secretary answered. I was crying so hard that I couldn't get my words out.

'It's OK,' she said, trying to calm me. 'Now tell me what's happened.'

'I'm a new mum and I'm still breastfeeding,' I stuttered. 'And I've got a lump. My doctor has just told me she's worried and is going to refer me, but I can't wait any longer. I've already had it for over three months. Please get Mr Williams to see me today.'

When I'd managed to get the rest of my story out – reiterating that my doctor was now really worried and how much time had passed since I'd first spotted the lump – the secretary kindly told me to drive straight there. The clinic was called the Spire.

'We'll try and get you in,' she promised.

Racing to the car, I was shaking so much I could hardly strap Gigi in. I just kept thinking, F***, what have I been waiting for? It's like a time-bomb waiting to go off inside me.

I rang Ash on the way, still crying hysterically.

'Please try and be calm, babe,' he told me. 'You don't know anything for sure yet. Why don't I jump in my car and come home so we can go together?'

But, from that moment on, I just wanted that lump out of me. Panic was tearing through my veins. I didn't have time to wait for Ash to meet up with me and take me there. Something had kicked in, and I knew that every second counted; I had to get to the clinic before I missed my opportunity to be seen. That was the most important thing.

'No, don't worry, Ash. You're so far away it could be ages before you get here. I'll just go straight there now and get seen.'

By the time I arrived at the Spire, I'd managed to compose myself a little.

The secretary at the front desk instructed me to fill in some forms and then asked me to take a seat. I sat there, biting my lip and rocking Gigi and praying over and over in my mind, and playing out every scenario in my head. I wasn't going anywhere until I'd been called, and I was in to see the consultant within the hour.

Mr Williams was a lovely man, very self-assured and composed, but he didn't believe in mincing his words.

'I'm very suspicious,' he told me bluntly.

The nightmare had begun.

That day, Mr Williams set the wheels in motion and, after a week and a half of being prodded and poked, I'd been given the most horrendous news: that, at the age of thirty-five, I had an aggressive form of breast cancer. I was no longer able to breastfeed my daughter and was taking bromcriptine to dry up my milk. Instead of enjoying those first few vital months with Gigi, the precious memories of her first gurgle, giggle or smile, I would be enduring a lumpectomy, chemotherapy and radiotherapy, and staring my own mortality in the face.

All of a sudden, life had never seemed bleaker . . .

6. The Fight Is On

It was an odd feeling, waking up the morning after I had been officially diagnosed with cancer.

As usual, it was Gigi's hungry cries that forced me out of bed, at 6.30 a.m. For a minute, as I stumbled to tend to her before she really started screaming, I couldn't quite recall why there was such a sinking feeling in my heart. Then the cogs in my brain whirled into action, reminding me with a jolt.

Oh God, I've got cancer, I thought. It's really happening.

Lots of people I have spoken to agree that the initial diagnosis is one of the worst parts of the whole thing. It's as if you draw a line under the life you have known up until that moment, kiss it goodbye and start all over again as a different person. Nothing is the same after that moment when you find out for definite. When you are first told, you don't know all the ins and outs of what's to come, all the different ways that things could play out, that as many people survive as die. All your everyday worries and little moans evaporate and a deep, deep fear takes root.

And it never really leaves. You know that your body

makes cancer and – even if it's caught early and treated successfully – there's always the thought that it could come back. It's like living on red alert. The diagnosis marks the beginning of a need to live day by day, making it through each one bringing a sense of utter relief.

In the hours and days that followed, it was as if the knowledge that I had cancer was playing on a loop in my head. I'd be making a cup of tea, or putting the washing out, and then it would pop into my mind and cause my stomach to lurch. 'It's only little,' I kept telling myself. 'It's a little lump and, soon, it'll be gone.'

It was strange, as at that point I didn't feel ill; in fact, I looked and felt great. I was someone who always had loads of energy, and I couldn't envisage being any other way. I'm going to get up every morning and give my daughter her bottle and a cuddle, no matter how tough it gets, I vowed. Without fail, I need to be her mum.

Knowing what I do now, I'm glad I had no idea how much of a struggle keeping that promise would be! There were mornings when I just wanted to curl up and disappear because of the side effects of my chemotherapy, times that I couldn't imagine fighting another day. But, with Gigi there, that was never really an option.

I've always been known for being very loud and chatty, but coming to terms with the news I had cancer left me feeling frightened and withdrawn. For the first time ever, other than my brief bout of baby blues, I became quite insular. I couldn't cope with interacting with lots of different people. I just wanted to cocoon myself in a bubble with Ash and shut out the world. He was my whole support system.

We stumbled through those first few dismal days, both in tears all the time.

Seeing Ash cry was just awful. I'd catch him sobbing, absolutely heartbroken. Before cancer entered our lives, I'd probably seen him cry only a handful of times in the sixteen years I'd known him. To see him so gutted, so scared, just killed me. And I couldn't stop crying. Every time I looked at Gigi, it set me off – I kept thinking back to those memory boxes I'd prepared as a legacy for my unborn baby. I had wanted to have my things in order, but I didn't imagine I'd need to have it done so soon.

My parents both immediately offered to come and stay, but I asked them not to for a while, which they understood and respected. I needed to get my head round everything that was happening, and I needed them to do the same, on their own. I couldn't carry their fear too, I needed to concentrate on me, Ash and Gigi. I couldn't cope with the thought of us all sitting around morbidly and waiting for the next person to burst into tears, or going through the ordeal of pretending it wasn't happening by discussing what to have for dinner or what was going on in the world – discussing anything except what was happening to us all, to me. That fake jollity people use to mask a nightmare situation wasn't something I could deal with at that point.

I knew Mum was really struggling to come to terms with the news, but it hit my dad hard too. I think he felt lost and helpless that he couldn't make it all OK for his little girl. There was no kissing this better; it was out of everyone's control. The week I found out, Dad's wife, Angie, was away visiting her family, so he was on his own. His sister lived near by, and I had to ring her to make sure he would be looked after until Angie got back. I didn't want him brooding on his own, full of worry, with no one to talk to. It's funny how things change, isn't it? Once I had Gigi, I realized that we all had very equal roles: my parents don't just parent me; it works the other way, too.

It's only a recent thing. When I did *Casualty*, I was constantly on the M5, going from Bristol to Devon to get my Mummy fix. After the stresses and strains of filming, I'd go home and collapse for a few days, and Mum would take over, look after me and sort out everything. But having a baby, never mind cancer, changes all that. Now I'm a mother, those natural urges to nurture and protect the people I love have kicked in with gusto.

As much as having cancer makes me feel like a frightened sixteen-year-old, it has also made me grow up. It's awakened an instinct to stand on my own two feet and accept responsibility for myself and my own family.

In a way, I also wanted to shield my parents from the worst of it. I hated worrying and upsetting them. All I'd ever wanted was to make them proud. I didn't factor in being diagnosed with a potentially terminal illness – it's not exactly one for the scrap book, is it? It's weird to be told you have something as massive as cancer, it unleashes all sorts of questions, the main ones being: Could I have done anything to avoid it? Have I done anything to cause it? – as well as the obvious one: Why me? I would look at Gigi and not be able to imagine my lovely daughter breaking the same news to me – how utterly desperate and helpless must you feel as a parent in that situation? You can't do the very thing that every parent instinctively wants to do: you can't take it away, you can't swap places and you can't remove the fear.

I had no idea what was going to be thrown at me during each stage of my experience, so I decided it was better to weather the storm at each turn and then tell my parents things slowly and gently, on a need-to-know basis.

Although Mum and I are really close, I didn't actually tell her about the lump until my third visit to the doctor's. She was sixty-five when it all happened and, although that is not old by any stretch of the imagination, I don't tend to ring her with the really worrying things any more. I think it's got something to do with me having a solid partner, too – it's a natural progression to confide in and be supported by the person you have made a life with. Ash is always my first port of call. That's what being in a long-term relationship does for you – it's all about building your own life and taking responsibility. It's definitely an age thing, too. When you're in your twenties, you ring your mum about every little thing, especially the stuff that goes wrong. But when Ash and I moved in together, it felt normal to stop burdening my mum and her partner Alan with stuff. I'd discuss it over dinner with Ash, or at our 'board meetings'. It was about us now.

If I'm honest about it, one of the things that stopped me telling Mum straight away was because I was also dealing with my own embarrassment – at having the lump in the first place, at not pursuing things with the doctor when I felt uneasy despite the all clear, and at finding a lump in my breast while heavily pregnant with her grandchild. Why couldn't I be like every other daughter and first-time mother and just feel great, look glowing and enjoy that special time? Let my mum enjoy her first grandchild?

In any case, I didn't tell her until I felt I really had to – once I was going to see the consultant, once I knew it was serious. Even then, I was reluctant. Mum had lost her sister Mary to breast cancer the previous April and had another friend my age who was currently losing her battle against the disease. For breast cancer already to have blighted her life so badly was more than she deserved. Why should she have to cope with the news that her daughter might have it too?

When I told her, I could tell she found it very overwhelming but, good old Mum, she stayed strong for me. We didn't discuss the fact that Aunty Mary had lost her

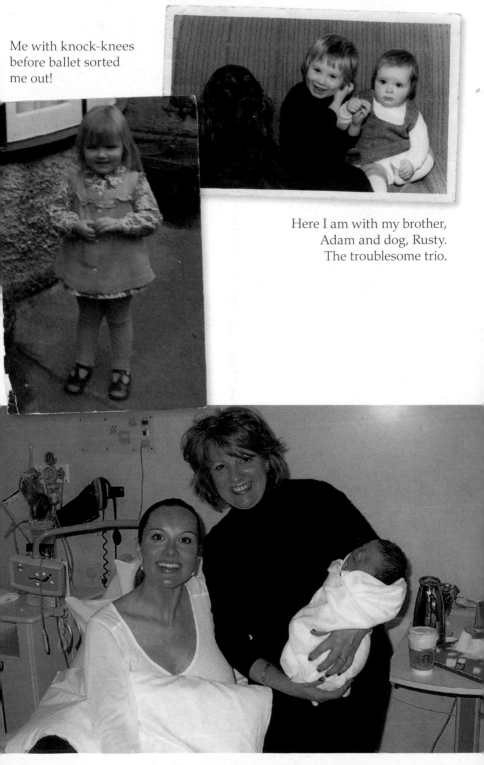

Me with knock-knees before ballet sorted me out!

Here I am with my brother, Adam and dog, Rusty. The troublesome trio.

Three generations. I've just given birth, but the lip gloss is in place!

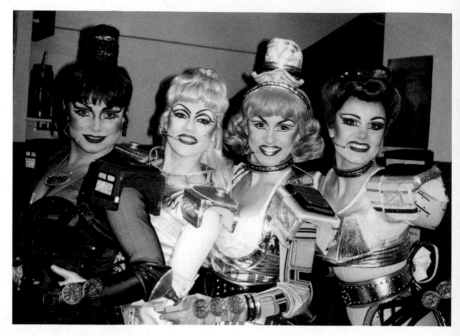

In *Starlight Express* with one of my dearest friends, Sam Lane, (far left). She has been a great support throughout my cancer battle.

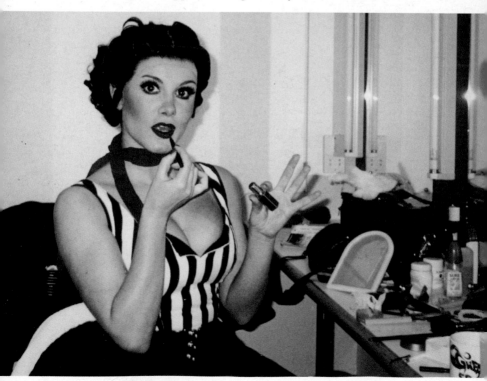

Me as Rizzo.

Beginning my career with the fabulous Bonnie Langford.

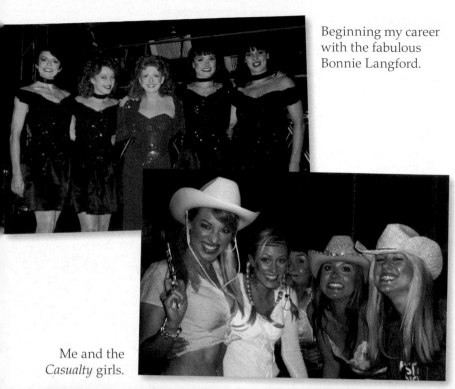

Me and the *Casualty* girls.

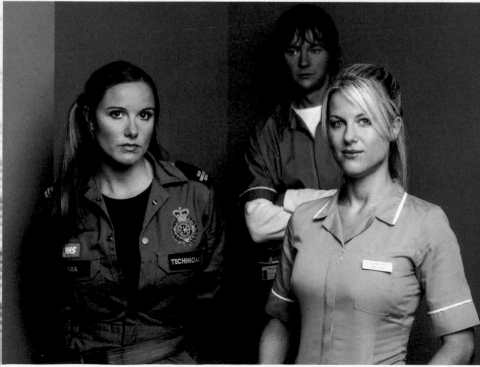

My Casualty love triangle with James Redmond and Georgina Bouzova.

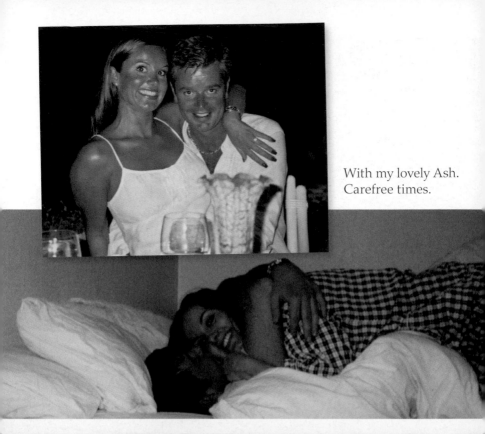

With my lovely Ash.
Carefree times.

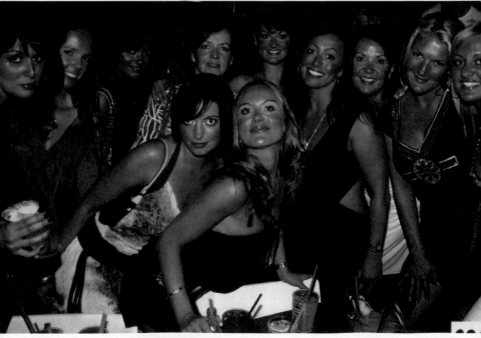

In Italy with the Torquay posse keeping the fake tan industry in business.

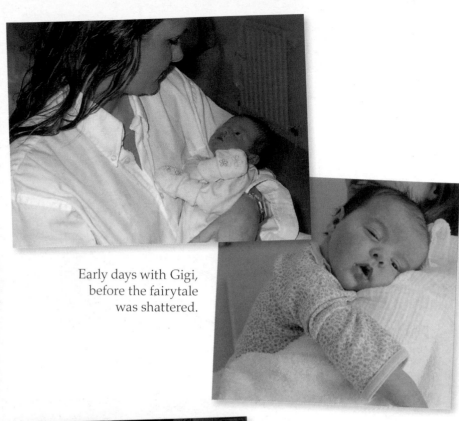

Early days with Gigi,
before the fairytale
was shattered.

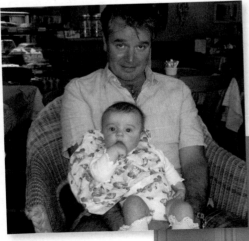

Daddy's Girl.

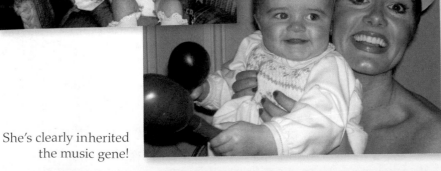

She's clearly inherited
the music gene!

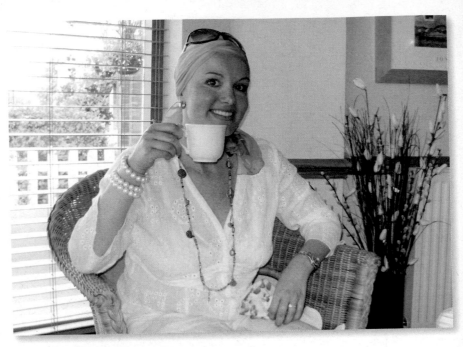

Determined to keep smiling through the sickness.

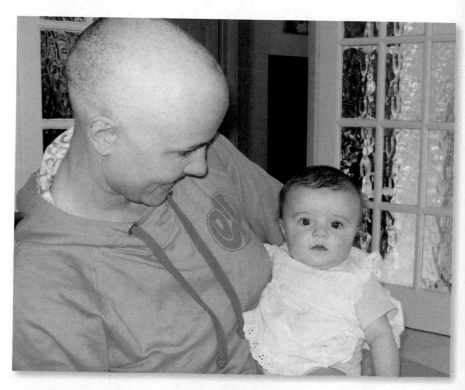

Just lost my hair, but Gigi still makes me smile.

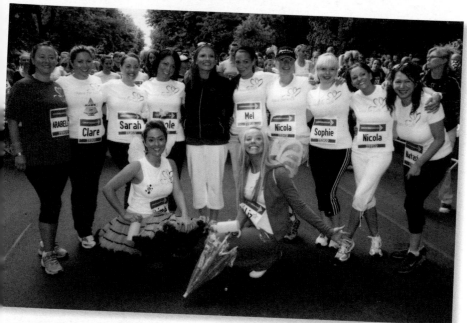

Ready to start the race for life.

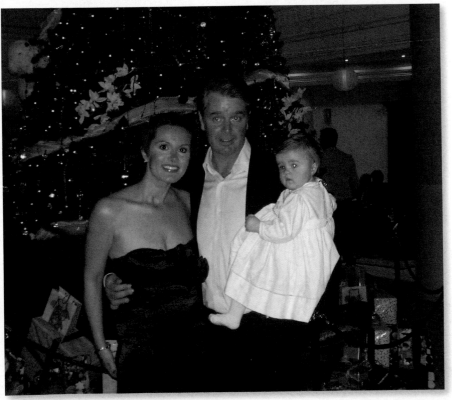

New Year's Eve 2008. We did it!

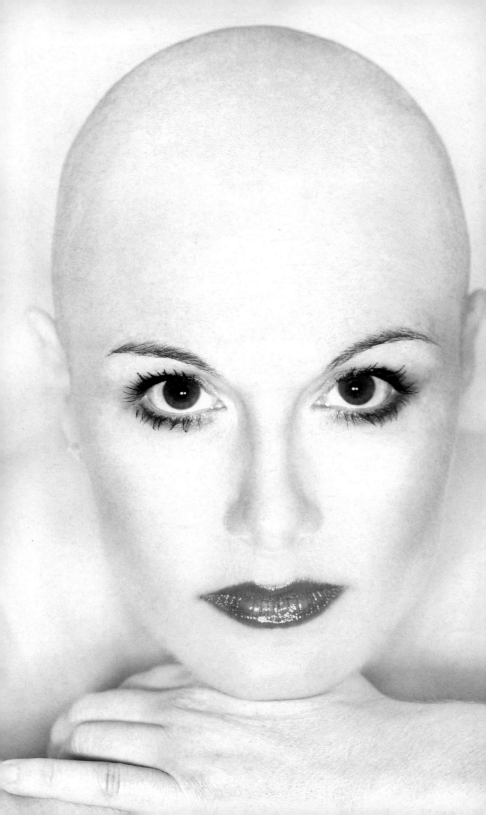

fight, or the fact that it might be genetic, I just didn't want to know about any of that – this had to be about me. I know now that, behind the scenes, Mum was having terribly low moments. She had the 3 a.m. fear but, thankfully, her partner, Alan, has been incredibly supportive of her, as have her friends.

'I find it very hard when people stop me in the street to console me,' she admitted to me during a heart-to-heart once I'd actually been diagnosed and she did come to stay. 'I get overwhelmed and break down.'

Which, if you know my mum, is not like her at all. She's an old-school lady – very proud and stiff upper lip. I think I have only heard her cry once, and that was when she was going through the divorce. When I was younger, I sometimes wished that she could be more demonstrative, that she found it easier to show her emotions, but I always knew she loved me.

Mum isn't one to weep and wail, she's tough and strong in a crisis, and has looked after me through a lot of low points whilst I fought the cancer. She'll come up for a week and take over – she'll be there cooking and getting on with it and making everything nice and jolly. She'll be sorting out hearty meals, looking after the baby and generally spreading some angel dust around the house.

But I wasn't prepared to sit there torturing her with my bleakest thoughts and worries. I just wasn't going to burden her with the truth when I was having a moment, or when I woke up in the night sweating and shaking at the prospect of a slow, painful death. No, my darkest fears and 'why me?' moments would be shared with Ash, and Ash alone. I decided right when it all started that he'd be my confidant from beginning to end and, as each difficult day panned out, I knew our love would grow stronger.

Thinking back to all those times now makes me feel very emotional. I've always enjoyed being in the limelight but, at that time, I was suddenly centre stage for all the wrong reasons. Cancer has such an effect on everyone, and they react so differently. I've had people cry and wail; others deflect the doom and gloom with astonishingly inappropriate jokes; and a few simply change the subject. One reaction that was general, though, was complete shock, because I was only thirty-five.

'Not you – you're so young, so fit and healthy,' people would say to me. 'How come?'

They needed answers, and I didn't have any. All I knew was that I was one of just twelve cases in my age group to have breast cancer in my whole healthcare trust. There was no rhyme or reason why this had happened to me. As healthy lifestyles went, mine was up there. I loved exercising and going swimming. When I worked in Bristol on *Casualty*, I was a member of a really nice gym with an outdoor pool. In the summer I'd be there at six every morning, splashing around, then I'd be on set at eight, raring to go, all bright-eyed and bushy-tailed.

I did smoke once upon a time, but I hadn't had a puff in years. And I didn't really drink much either – apart from the odd glass of champagne now and then over the past eight years, I've been pretty much dry. Hardly a hedonistic lifestyle!

I'd even inspired Ash to give up the booze.

Not long after we met, he had asked me why I didn't drink, and I told him, 'Because I'm high on life!' I think he really liked that. 'It was one of the endearing things that made me fall in love with you,' he now says, and it wasn't long after that that he gave up too.

We've always eaten well, too – lots of fresh fruit and veg and not too much red meat. My health obsession even went so far as trying to get Ash to give up his beloved Diet Coke. I limited him to one can at the weekend (although I'm sure when I'm not there he has about five).

But none of my precautions and healthy ways had saved me. You can do all the virtuous living in the world, but cancer can still strike, as I'd discovered. It's a simple bloody lottery, and it was terrifying. My friends were amazing, the way they rallied round, but it was so close to home for one of the group to be diagnosed with something so frightening, especially when we were all of a similar age. I think that's why my girlfriends bombarded me with questions – if they could find the reason I had it, then it somehow made more sense. It made them feel safer to be able to point to something that had happened in my life as 'the cause'. It made the hideous disease less indiscriminate and less uncontrollable.

Right from the start, I'd made it very clear that I wanted to have the lumpectomy done privately. I wanted the guarantee that I'd have Mr Williams doing the operation. He'd treated my friend Madeleine really well, and I'd liked him straight away and felt safe in his care.

But, although I had complete faith in my consultant, I did seek out another opinion. It wasn't that I didn't trust Mr Williams, but being misdiagnosed twice had left me feeling very insecure. I just wanted to make absolutely sure.

The day I went for that other opinion, I was cramming a lot in.

In the morning, I was finally taking Gigi for her very late six-week check-up. (We'd delayed it because of our holiday in Spain and then once more because it clashed with a hospital appointment.) I needed to be there for 9.15 a.m. And, on the way there, in a moment of positive thinking, I had prayed to the parking fairies for an easy space to leave my car in.

When I drove up, I was thrilled to see the perfect spot, with plenty of room to manoeuvre Gigi out of the car. It was even illuminated by a beam of sunshine. The parking fairies had delivered!

I had just pulled into the pavement to reverse into the space when, out of nowhere, a twentysomething lad in his souped-up wagon came flying round the corner and nicked it.

Without a moment's thought, I shot out of my car and raced over to him, crying uncontrollably. 'I've got f***ing breast cancer,' I shrieked, my voice high-pitched with hysteria. 'I'm now going to be late for a baby check that was already four weeks overdue, and a second opinion in London, as I no longer trust ANYONE, including YOU, who just stole MY parking space!'

As I stood there, all red-faced and blotchy and shoulders shaking, the lad looked at me like I was a madwoman, his face pale and full of shock. Then he put his car into reverse and screeched off.

Wiping my eyes and sniffing, I turned to look at Gigi, who was sitting in her car seat, contentedly chewing on her thumb. She was gazing at me with a look that said, 'What is my crazy mummy doing?' But crazy Mummy got her parking space and made it to the appointment on time.

After the breast-cancer diagnosis had brought my world crashing down, I was, understandably, going through a stage where I was always expecting the unexpected. So, pushing Gigi's pram into the baby clinic, I couldn't begin to imagine how I'd cope if something was up with her as well.

Thankfully, after a thorough examination, all my fears were dispelled. Gigi passed her six-week check with flying colours, and any worries I had turned out to be completely unfounded.

As we were leaving, I looked at a text I'd received that day from Sue Packer, my old *Casualty* castmate. 'Enjoy what there is to enjoy,' it read. So I did, and phoned Ash excitedly. Gigi's clean bill of health was definitely something to celebrate.

That afternoon, I trekked into London for the further opinion on my treatment, which I'd organized via my antenatal consultant at the Portland.

When I'd called the consultant's secretary and explained my predicament, she'd quickly arranged for me to see a very respected doctor who came highly recommended. Twenty years earlier, he'd been instrumental in a real breakthrough, which had led to pioneering surgery in which lymph glands were removed from breast-cancer sufferers to help stop the disease spreading.

Going back to the Portland for such an awful reason was unbelievably sad. I'd spent so much time there, leading up to Gigi's birth. It had been such an exciting thing in my life and I'd got to know lots of the staff really well. I dreaded going back there for this.

After Gigi was born, I'd promised I'd come back and visit the staff with her. But, instead of enjoying people cooing over my baby, I was sitting in Outpatients without her (she was at home with Ash) and feeling miserable. I'd kept my head down going in, as I didn't want to see anyone. I just wasn't ready to tell them what was happening to me, to see their shocked looks or hear the sympathy in their voices.

I should be here showing off my baby, not sitting here waiting to talk about cancer and death, I thought sadly as, yet again, it hit me that the ideal family life I'd envisaged was slipping through my fingers. Thankfully, my maudlin moment was interrupted by a nurse calling me in to see Professor Baum.

'So, how can I help you today, Rebekah?' he asked, greeting me.

'I have every faith in the NHS and my consultant,' I explained nervously, 'but I wondered if you would be willing to read my notes and examine me, just to make sure everything is being handled correctly?' I continued, 'You see, I was told twice it was a milk duct, so I have had a lump for nearly four months, and now I've been told it's cancer. I'm just feeling worried about everything.'

After he'd examined me, Professor Baum flicked through the notes that had been made on my case to date. Finally, he spoke, confirming Mr Williams' diagnosis but giving me some room for hope: yes, it was definitely cancer, but he was 100 per cent sure that everything was in place for my recovery; we were going for a cure and, now I was in the system, I would be taken care of. I felt ready for the fight now. I was totally sure I was on the right track, that I knew what I was dealing with.

'Mr Williams is an excellent doctor,' he told me warmly.

'Thank you,' I said, smiling gratefully.

Leaving that room, for the first time since my diagnosis,

I felt upbeat about my treatment. Professor Baum's words had given me hope and strength. Suddenly, the whole thing didn't seem so daunting. I was in safe hands, and I felt I had as good a chance as any of beating it.

After that, the week or so leading up to the operation, seemed very full. I was doing my research, talking to people and I was treating it all with the enthusiasm and hard work I'd throw into a job (just like when I was pregnant with Gigi). I was going all out to make sure everything was covered, to ensure I had all the facts, and generally giving it 100 per cent positivity. It helped to be so busy and pro-active. But in reality I was falling to pieces.

Sue, the cancer-specialist nurse from the Kent and Sussex hospital, had been liaising with her counterpart, a nurse called Maggie, at Spire Healthcare in Tunbridge Wells, and explained to me that she would be my first port of call for the operation. So, the Thursday before my surgery, I went in to see Maggie for a pre-operation check-up.

That day, my positive thinking was taking a pounding, and I'd woken up in the worst mood. It was a real 'why me?' day, and I felt irrationally angry at everything and everyone. Well, I guess it wasn't really that irrational – in truth, I wasn't getting much sleep and I felt totally exhausted. I was sick to death of all the toing and froing to hospital and, on top of it all, boy, was Gigi grouchy too.

I kept wondering why, but then it dawned on me that she must be picking up on my stress levels. This poor little girl had had absolute calm in her life and, now, she had a mum who was all over the place, who didn't know whether to laugh or cry.

Instantly, I felt guilty for being a bad mother – and that made me even more crabby and upset. I felt like such a failure – and I really took it out on Ash. He couldn't do a thing right. If he wanted to come to appointments with me, I accused him of fussing; if he didn't offer, I would tell him that he didn't care enough. When he tried to help with Gigi, I would tell him he wasn't doing it in the right way; when he didn't take her, I'd accuse him of leaving it all to me. He just couldn't win. Those bleak days before the operation were hard on both of us. It was such a scary time. We'd had no preparation for this new world we were inhabiting, we hadn't asked to be here, and we were both petrified.

I was still doing my best to be upbeat in front of my daughter but, whenever I gazed at her asleep, looking so small and vulnerable in her cot, it just floored me. It tore my heart in two to think I might not be there to see her grow up.

If there's one thing I've learned about cancer, it's that you never know how you're going to feel when you wake up in the morning, let alone hour to hour and minute to minute. One day you'll be happy, the next you'll be sad. It's like riding a rollercoaster – heady highs of optimism followed by dark dips of despair – but it's all part of the experience. You just have to learn to go with the flow.

One morning, just before the operation, I'd popped to the supermarket to pick up a few essentials.

As I meandered up and down the aisle with Gigi, I wasn't in too bad a mood, and I'd temporarily forgotten my affliction. It was nice to feel as if I was a normal mum wandering around the supermarket with my baby, pondering over nothing more taxing than whether to buy leek and potato soup or carrot and coriander. Then I saw her – Alex, a friend of a friend – heading down the aisle towards me, her forehead crinkled in concern. Oh God, here we go, I thought, with a sinking feeling.

'Rebekah, how *are* you?' she asked when she reached me. 'I was *so* sorry to hear your news.'

'Oh you know,' I stammered awkwardly. 'I'm fine. Bearing up. What can you do?'

Cue five minutes of uncomfortable chat. Again. As I said goodbye, all hope of being a normal civilian for an hour was lost, and I felt as if the words 'CANCER VICTIM' were back stamped on my forehead.

I really hated the fact that I was feeling so negative towards someone who had been sweet enough to come and ask how I was doing, to ask after my wellbeing – but, at that point, every time someone asked how things were going, it felt like the knife was being twisted.

Later, as I was getting ready to travel to the hospital for my appointment with Maggie, it felt like the biggest effort. My home was my little haven, and I resented having to get myself organized to leave it. I should be here worrying about Gigi's next feed, not going off to talk about bloody cancer, I thought crossly as I piled nappies, bottles and wet wipes into her travel bag.

Thankfully, Victoria, my neighbour, had offered to come to the hospital with me to look after Gigi. Throughout my illness, she has been a pillar of strength. She'll just turn up on the doorstep with a home-cooked lasagne or a crate of Lucozade. She really knows how to mother me, and just when I need it.

When I started the chemo, she even did my washing and my shopping for me – anything she could do to help. But I think the best thing she ever did while I was having treatment was come to the rescue one day when I was changing my bedlinen. I felt particularly wretched and thought how nice it would be to have a nap in luxurious clean sheets, so I stripped the bed and set about making it up. All of a sudden, I just couldn't carry on. All the strength had gone out of my body, and I felt as if I was going to be violently ill. I called Victoria, and in she came – in an instant, she had finished the bed and put me firmly in it. She even washed and ironed the old sheets. It set the pattern for a weekly luxury, and I couldn't thank her enough for it.

The generosity and kindness of people such as Victoria who, ultimately, owe me nothing, as I have battled my cancer stage by stage, has never ceased to amaze me. It sounds like a cliché, but an illness like this really does underline who your real friends are. Those who stick around after the initial shock of the diagnosis has worn off, after you've had the operation and treatment but are still haunted by those black thoughts of it coming back, when you feel unbelievably exhausted and sad that this has happened to you – those friends are priceless.

Ash's mum, Jen, has been incredible, too. If I had to go to hospital, she was always on hand to take the baby at a moment's notice. She was always strong around me and really understood that I needed practical support rather than lots of sympathetic looks and tears. I know she was a fantastic help to Ash too – sometimes I just couldn't deal with his fear on top of everything else, I couldn't be there for him in the way he was used to me being. Ash has always said that one of the things that helped him fall in love with me was how caring and giving I was, but it wasn't always easy to be that way – especially when faced with my own mortality.

It helped that Ash was still working in the run-up to the operation, as we needed the money. When you've got your own business, nobody else can share the burden, make the decisions or do the books. Ash didn't have any choice but to work. He'd had four days off during my diagnosis period, but the business couldn't afford for him to take much more. I also suspect that immersing himself in work helped him to stay sane. For me, it was a relief that he had something to keep him occupied. I needed to be selfish.

Yet we were still nowhere near the end. We knew I still faced a long road. I'd had the initial scan, I'd taken the medication to dry up my milk, I'd had to get Gigi used to formula – but there would be more scans, and I needed to have a lumpectomy, I had to prepare myself for some kind of treatment afterwards, and perhaps even more bad news if the cancer had spread. I had to gear up mentally for a hard slog, and it felt like the whole thing was a bottomless pit of horror. At this point, Ashley's mother became like my second mum. She lived so near by, I would just go round to hers, hand her the baby and get some sleep. At other times, we'd just have cups of tea and biscuits, and she'd tell me, 'This will define you, this will make you a stronger person.'

Right from the beginning, Jen has hammered home that Ash and I are strong, that we could cope with this. The truth is that, when I found out I had cancer, I had no faith whatsoever in my strength. The fact that friends, and family like Jen, believed I had the stamina to survive helped to make me feel and be able to think positively. When you are facing the unthinkable, you need inspiring, strong and focused people in your life and, without Jen and Victoria, I'm not sure how I would have coped.

However, going back to that particular day, as we travelled across town in the car for my pre-op appointment, Victoria was to see me at my worst.

By the time she called round to accompany me, I'd already worked myself up into a total frenzy. I'm quite embarrassed when I think back now, but I couldn't stop once I'd started, and I ranted and raged all the way to the hospital.

'I'm the frigging healthiest person I know!' I seethed. 'I go to the gym all the time! My grandmother had breast cancer in her eighties, but I'm only thirty-five! What the hell have I done to deserve this sh*t?'

I raged on and on, so angry about the dodgy card fate had dealt me, spitting out every nasty swearword I could think of until, inevitably, the tears came, and I cried and cried.

'I'm sorry, Victoria,' I sobbed. 'But it's just so bloody unfair.'

Bless Victoria, she was brilliant.

She listened without interrupting, and then did her best to soothe me. There weren't any answers, I knew that, but it felt good to unleash a bit of my fear and frustration on someone I knew I didn't have to be strong for. Once we'd arrived at the hospital, I'd managed to regain my composure a bit.

But, while Maggie the nurse was perfectly lovely, it still took every ounce of self-restraint I had to sit there and be courteous and polite.

Maggie took my blood pressure, listened to my heart and did a blood test. 'You'll have to wear a loose bra after the operation,' she told me, indicating a pile of bland fawn brassieres in the corner of the room. 'And we need to monitor the drain site from your surgery wound carefully to make sure it doesn't get infected.'

The conversation that followed – about physio, allergies and button-at-the-front clothing – made me feel furious. I didn't know what had come over me, but I was consumed by rage. I forced myself to nod and show willing but, inside, I'd regressed to being a moody teenager and was sat there thinking, 'Yeah, whatever! I don't want to be here, love!'

Maggie carried on diligently, gently telling me the protocol . . . how I'd arrive at 7 a.m., that I couldn't eat for twelve hours beforehand, that I'd probably be in hospital for three days, depending on how the surgery went . . . But I could hear Gigi crying outside, and I was barely listening. Yep, yep, where do I sign? I thought impatiently. Get me out of here. Then, as if we were psychically linked – and at exactly the moment I felt ready to explode – I heard Gigi letting out an ear-piercing scream of frustration.

I took a deep breath and smiled at Maggie. It wasn't her fault, but she was in the firing line. I consoled myself with the fact that she must have seen this a million times over – tears, rage, disbelief: the works. Hers wasn't exactly the jolliest of jobs. I don't know how people deal with a job like that, where every day brings another round of heartbreak.

Somehow, I managed to get through the rest of the appointment, taking notes, as I knew Ash would have loads of questions when he got home from work later. I tried to ask sensible questions and get as much information as I could while Victoria paced the corridor with Gigi. In the end, I felt better for having gone, and for being a little more informed about what was about to happen to me. But knowing more didn't make me like any of it. That's what you soon come to realize about cancer: it's not just a lump – that's just the beginning of the whole mini-series of hell; and I didn't want to know anything about any of it. It was almost like, if I refused to acknowledge it, to let it into my perfect world, then it couldn't hurt me.

Back home later, I cried and swore some more, then set about cleaning and vigorously hoovering the house before flopping on the sofa, too exhausted to feel angry and aggressive any more.

Nothing will change by Wednesday, it's going to happen, I thought to myself. I'm going to have to get used to it. I just need to focus on what I can do to make it better.

I planned lots of girlie catch-ups to take my mind off everything. I didn't want any time on my hands to think about what was coming. In the few days before the op, though, Ash asked me not to go haring around the M25 to see my girlfriends.

'I want you to rest,' he told me. 'You're going to need all the strength you can get, Becks. Go for some nice walks and get some fresh air.'

So I went to see Alison, who lived down the road from me in Tonbridge. She'd just had a knee op, and some of our other old friends from college were there, too. It felt just like old times. We ate biscuits and drank tea, and they laughed as I told them about my psycho episode in the car park.

Everyone was being really careful not to mention the cancer and the fact I was about to go in for an op – I guess people don't know what to say – but Alison always uses humour to diffuse an awkward situation, so she cracked a joke about how she and Maria could run a marathon with my name on their vests. I immediately took it the wrong way – weren't charity runs usually done to raise money for people who had died? Yet again, I was full of anger. I'm not f***ing dead yet! I thought.

It took a lot of self-control not to totally lose it there and then, but everyone could tell that I was upset, the atmosphere changed in an instant, and I left soon after. I couldn't trust myself not to blow up, and I knew it would make me feel worse. I didn't know what was happening to me – I was so irrational.

Alison had obviously only meant to distract me and lighten the situation, but no one could win with me at the time. I was laughing one minute and weeping the next, I was so volatile. I think back now and feel really sorry for my friends and Ash.

One of the things I found hardest was dealing with other people's reaction to my illness. When friends called me up and burst into tears, it was me who had to console them, which could be draining, even though I knew they were just reacting from the heart. Yet I always preferred those friends who addressed what was going on rather than those who ignored it, out of embarrassment.

For me, personally, the nights were by far the worst time. I'd lie awake torturing myself, imagining all the different scenarios the future could hold. I might not be around to see Gigi's second birthday, let alone her twenty-first, I'd think morbidly. It made my heart race and my throat tighten with emotion. How could my little girl grow up without her mummy? It was always Mum who had done all the small things that were so important when I was young, like tying my shoelaces, kissing my bruised knee after a tumble, or rubbing my belly better if I felt poorly.

I could still recall that anxious knot in my tummy when I smelt her perfume and understood that she was going out for the evening – and I could still remember stirring sleepily but being instantly comforted when a gentle kiss on my forehead told me she was home once more and I could rest safe and sound.

Not that I could be sad for too long. Every moment with Gigi was an absolute joy. Just that week, she'd developed a dirty little laugh, which just cracked me up. Looking at her sitting in her bouncy chair next to the window, I would think, God, I love that girl.

Packing the day before the op was a nightmare. As well as gathering together everything I'd need for my hospital visit, I had to pack for the baby, who was going to stay with Jen.

I'd specifically asked Ash to stay at his mum and dad's for those three days I would be away. The thought of him going home on his own upset me; I knew he wouldn't eat properly. He'd need his mum to look after him, and I needed to know my babies were safe.

I'd never been away from Gigi overnight, and the thought of it was daunting. Even the logistics of packing bogged me down. I spent the whole day preparing for her stay with Ash's mum, making sure Jen had all the necessaries – sterilizer, nappies and bottles; then there was the bedding, the travel cot, the baby-gros. I worried that Gigi wouldn't settle, as it was always me who did the nightshift. It was our special time together. I always loved tucking her up safely, leaving a light on and stroking her forehead as she drifted off to sleep. What if she wanted me in the night when I was in hospital? Wasn't it my job to be there for her?

The night before I went into hospital, as I was settling Gigi down, I realized I was using the prospect of three nights away from her as a distraction. The fact was, cancer could steal me from her for ever.

I already know instinctively what she needs, I thought to myself, watching her eyelids droop until she was sleeping peacefully. I know when she cries to be fed or just wants a hug. I know what she likes and what she doesn't. If I'm not here, who will smile at her in the morning?

Later, lying in bed, I managed to relax a bit by imagining all the fun things I was going to do to get me through the next few months. I cuddled up to Ash and recited what I had lined up for us. I'm going to go for walks with my baby, I decided. I'm going to make plans, go for nice lunches, have friends round, visit the theatre, sit in the garden and finally use my picnic hamper. I might even set a date for our wedding! I'm going to get up, shower and dress every day – and put my lipgloss on. No matter what, I'll paint on a smile.

Ash held me tight and said some lovely things to me, we had a cry, and then tried to get some sleep. Of course, I tossed and turned for most of the night, getting up repeatedly to check on Gigi and to watch her sleeping.

The next morning, I was up at 5 a.m., and decidedly uncheery.

I jumped in the shower, shaving under my arm, ready for the op, then dressed and dried my hair. I'd cleaned the house from top to bottom and had made it look all nice for our return, but I still ran round at least ten times checking everything was in its place.

'You're so OCD at times,' Ash chastised me, as I checked for the sixth time that the front door was locked.

Last, but not least, we placed Gigi in her car seat. She sat there grumpily, staring at Ziggy the zebra. No matter how hard I tried, I couldn't get a single smile out of her. She wasn't having anything to do with my silly faces and singing.

Ash drove us to his mum's in silence, neither of us daring to speak in case the tears came. He knew I didn't want Gigi seeing me all upset.

As we pulled up at Jen's house, I caught sight of my reflection in the mirror. I had my lippy on, but I was finding it hard to crack a smile. It was killing me to leave my baby but, bless Jen, she was raring to go and immediately set to work helping us unload all Gigi's stuff – the girl had more baggage than Paris Hilton! Giving her a last kiss and cuddle, I handed her over to Jen, with a warmed bottle.

'She's due a feed,' I told her, just about managing to hold it together.

Jen looked ecstatic at the thought of a three-day bonding session with her granddaughter. I was relieved that, now she had woken up a bit, Gigi was all smiles with Jen, and hadn't cried on me.

'She's in good hands,' I told myself as I clambered back in the car, biting my lip. We headed off in a daze. I sat silently next to Ash, trying not to cry, in a state of shock. I stared out of the window at the world rushing by. The streets were scattered with early-morning joggers and people walking their dogs, everyone going about their daily business, oblivious of my watching. Right then, I would have done anything to trade places with any of them.

We arrived at the clinic at about 7 a.m., and were taken straight to my room. I did the obligatory thing of getting my toiletries out, along with my perfume, then I turned on the telly to watch GMTV, desperate for some sense of normality.

A nurse came in and did all my checks, testing my blood pressure and my pulse. The whole thing gave me a weird sense of déjà vu – just three months earlier, I'd been in exactly the same situation, before giving birth to Gigi. But back then, though, I was full of nervous excitement. Today I was utterly petrified.

After a while, the anaesthetist popped in to explain his role, and then Mr Williams arrived. He asked how I was feeling and then talked about what would happen during my surgery.

'We'll remove the lump and take a good cut around it to check we have removed all the cancer,' he explained. 'We'll also remove your lymph glands and do tests to see if the cancer is in them, too.'

Ash could barely meet my eye, he was trying so hard to hold it all together. He knew he couldn't fall apart on me here.

When Mr Williams had gone, I changed into my hospital gown, ready for the operation. While we were waiting, I gazed out of the window at the gorgeous gardens. A beautiful morning was unfolding but, then, something black and white flew into my line of vision.

'That magpie!' I shrieked at Ash.

He raced to the window and looked at me in dismay as it started pecking around on the lawn. Surely it couldn't be the same sodding doom merchant who had been hanging around in our garden ever since my bad luck began?

'Look!' said Ash, as another bird landed on the lawn. 'Two magpies!'

We both grinned. Seeing two magpies was like we'd won the lottery. We were holding on to any little thing we could.

The week previously, my friend Georgina had come round and had accidentally stood on my home-made feng-shui frog (a three-legged amphibian with a Chinese coin in its mouth that symbolizes prosperity). I was gutted – until Mum quickly sent me a new one (as did a mortified Georgina later on). It was ridiculous but, when you are grasping at straws, anything that brings comfort helps.

As the countdown continued, I felt so nervous I was shaking. In true Ash style, he stepped up to the plate. He knew what he had to do, and he kept making me laugh, cracking jokes to take my mind off things. I don't know how he does it, but he always helps me to see the funny side when times are tough. Even just his smell as he hugged me brought me comfort. I've never needed anyone as much as I need him. I can't begin to comprehend how people cope when they have to go through it alone. I'm not sure I could.

When the time came for me to go down to theatre, Ash looked as apprehensive as I felt, so I tried to smile bravely, even though I felt like jelly inside.

'Be good, gorge!' he said (referring to the word I over-use the most), and then kissed me firmly on the forehead.

'I'll see you in a bit. And I'll be right here when you wake up.'

As they started to wheel me down to the operating theatre, I had an urge to jump off the bed and run away, but I knew I had no choice but to stay put.

'OK, Rebekah?' the anaesthetist asked, as he put in a line for the anaesthetic.

All I could do was nod. I knew if I tried to speak I would cry.

The liquid began to filter into my veins, and I stared at the clock and saw it was 8.17 a.m. The last thing I remember was an itchy feeling at the back of my throat; then there was nothing.

'OK, Beck?' Ash's voice seemed distant but, slowly, I began to stir.

After waking up in the recovery ward after the operation, I'd been drifting in and out of sleep. At some stage, the porter must have wheeled me back to my room, and I woke again, to the sound of Ash checking on me. I could also hear someone enthusiastically discussing interest rates and mortgages on the TV.

The time was 11.45 a.m., and Ash was there by my side. 'How are you feeling?' he asked gently.

'OK,' I said, trying my best to keep my eyelids open.

My head felt so heavy but, once I'd summoned up the strength, I took a moment to look down at my breast. Just before the operation, I'd signed a waiver to say that I gave permission for them to take further surgical action if they believed the cancer had spread. I knew there was a small chance I could have had more taken away than I had expected. But, through the bandaging, I could just about see that, despite some swelling and a tube where the drain site was, all was still intact.

Feeling exhausted, but relieved, I put my head back down again. It was a wonderful feeling to be able to just float off. The next time I woke up, it was 3 p.m.

'Your phone has been going all day,' Ash smiled. 'You've had nineteen text messages!'

Ash had popped home to his mum's while I was under. I'd asked him not to bring Gigi up to the hospital. 'It's no place for a baby,' I told him. Instead, he'd brought me video clips and photos of her on his phone. She looked so cute.

After I had regained my strength by drinking lots of water and tea and eaten some toast, Ash bid me goodbye to go home to Gigi. As the evening drew in, I took a temazepam to help me sleep and a couple of tramadol to ease the pain. I fell asleep thinking about my Gigi's gorgeous little face.

I was woken at 2 a.m. by a nurse coming in to check on me. All sleepy and a bit delirious, I forgot where I was and instinctively hissed, 'Sshhh, you'll wake her.' Then I wearily remembered that I wasn't at home with Ash, and there was no little angel at the bottom of my bed.

Despite missing my family, the following morning I awoke feeling optimistic. This is it, I've toughened up, I thought to myself. No more feeling sorry for myself. The scar under my arm was three inches long and really hurt, but it was good to think that that nasty little tumour was gone.

'It's all up from here, Becks,' Ash agreed. 'They've got the bad stuff out and, once you've recovered, they'll zap it to make sure it's all gone, and this whole thing will seem like a distant nightmare.'

I smiled in agreement. For the first time in weeks, I felt as if the black cloud was lifting. I was setting off on the road to recovery, and all was going to be well.

But, on my last day in hospital, I could sense that Ash was having a low moment. He seemed angry. Poor Ash. After his initial tears, he'd been trying so hard to be strong for me. But, in those bleak weeks, he had clearly felt completely cheated by fate, just as I had. He was a proud new father besotted with his lovely baby daughter and head over heels with his wife-to-be. Then, out of nowhere, his world had come crashing down.

As much as I'd tried to offer him support, he clearly hated to burden me with what he was really going through. I knew that his forty-minute drive to work each day gave him a lot of time to think, and to digest everything that was happening to us, but I did hope he was confiding in his friends too. Once the lump was out, it was as if I'd entered a new phase: only positive thoughts allowed. It was the only way I could cope.

What I didn't know was that there was a good reason for Ash's mood. After begging Mr Williams for information, he'd eventually been told that the cancer had probably invaded my lymph glands and he had decided not to tell me until the results came back and we knew for sure. He wanted me to concentrate on getting over the operation and then on being strong enough to face the next hurdle, so he carried the weight of that secret around for nine whole days – it must have felt like an eternity. God love that man of mine.

It was weird because, despite his mood and the constant frown, it was always Ash insisting that we had to be 100 per cent positive. If I did get weepy or start thinking 'what if', Ash would seize my hand, look me square in the eye and tell me insistently: 'There's no room for negativity.'

What we did ascertain after those first few days of crying was that there is actually nothing to be gained from tears. It doesn't change a thing, and you just end up feeling worse. Ash's stance was that we didn't know the facts, so there was no point pitying ourselves and thinking the worst.

Throughout this time, Ash was, and still is, extremely protective of me. I know now that he told everyone to remain as positive as possible around me. Even now, if anyone breaks down or starts being negative, he steps in and tells them they're not helping.

For example, when my mum came up from Devon just before I started chemotherapy, I started picking her brains about her friend Karen, who was my age and had terminal cancer, which had started off in her breast. Sadly, Karen has since passed away but, at the time of my diagnosis, doctors had given her a year to live, and she was having a life ceremony with all her family and friends.

Poor Mum, I knew she'd been to hell and back over my diagnosis. She must have felt plagued by breast cancer. She was still reeling after my Aunty Mary's death, her mother had battled the disease in her old age, her friend Karen wasn't going to make it, and now she was hoping and praying for her daughter too.

'When you first told me, I would have done anything to swap places with you,' she revealed. 'I thought, I've had my sixty-five years, it's me who should have the cancer, not my daughter, who has just had a baby of her own. I ached to make it better and step into your shoes. No mother should have to see her child suffer.'

But, despite my 'positive' stance, I couldn't help but probe deeper about Karen's cancer. Mum had accompanied her to chemo a few times and talked freely about it. As we drank tea in the front room, I was firing questions at her such as – 'What drug was she on? Herceptin? What grade did they say her cancer was? A morbid part of me needed to know, to weigh up the odds and work out my own chances.

But Ash didn't like it one bit. A little while later, he called

Mum into the kitchen. 'Please don't indulge her. She doesn't need to hear details like that, it's not good for her,' he said.

For Ash to be like this was surprising. He'd never been confrontational before or stepped in with my friends or family. But his steadfast belief that we had to stay positive was clearly overriding his usual politeness. Plus, he knew that the road ahead wasn't going to be an easy one now that the cancer had spread.

'It's so vital for you to be upbeat, Becks,' he said to me that evening. 'What can ever be achieved by being anything else?'

So, when a beaming Ash came to collect me on the Saturday after my op (I'd been examined by Mr Williams, who seemed pleased with my progress and had given me the all clear to go home), he was clearly taking some of his own advice.

When he walked in the door, I was already packed and waiting to go – and I was so relieved to see his mood had lightened. 'Take me home, please!' I grinned.

In the car, travelling first to Jen's, I was beside myself with excitement at the prospect of seeing my Gigi. As soon as we arrived at the house, I hurried upstairs to her room. My little angel was fast asleep and looked so peaceful that I didn't have the heart to pick her up and wake her. Instead, I wafted my perfume over her, to see if that would stir her, but she was clearly out for the count.

When Gigi finally woke up, it was amazing. I was in agony from my surgery, but nothing was going to stop me from cuddling her. I'd only had my drain taken out of the wound that morning, so it was pretty painful. My movement was limited, and the physiotherapist had told me I might never get the full range back. It was an alien feeling to be so inactive and feel so restricted.

Picking Gigi up made me wince, but it was lovely to embrace her, and I felt very emotional. Even in three days, she'd changed so much.

'Hello, little one,' I cooed. 'Mummy missed you.'

My first night at home didn't go quite as smoothly as planned. I'd been told to keep checking my dressing and that, if I noticed that the discharge from the wound went at all yellowy in colour, I would need to have it re-dressed.

Well, Sod's law, when it got to nine o'clock that Saturday night, I could see all this blood mixed in with yellow discharge on the wound. I couldn't re-dress it myself, because of the limited movement in my arm, and I didn't really want Ash to do it, so I rang up the hospital, and they told me to come in.

I wasn't able to drive myself, so it meant that all three of us had to venture out into the cold, so that Ash could drive.

On the way, I looked at Gigi, all sleepy and grouchy in her car seat, and thought, Oh God, there's so much more to this than I could ever have imagined. It's going to affect every corner of our lives. I was feeling tired and tearful from the operation and, at that moment, I just felt physically and mentally exhausted.

Of course, once we got there, a nurse was quickly able to clean up and re-dress my wound with no problem but, by the time we got home at 10.30 p.m., I felt drained.

That night, while Ash was downstairs and Gigi was sleeping, I lay in bed and had a cry. This is what my life is going to be like from now on, I thought. Endless hospital visits and anxiety. Everything else I've worried about in the past seems so insignificant compared to this. This is the whole package, this is what you get with cancer.

It was relentless, I just couldn't see a light at the end of the tunnel. It was completely overwhelming. Cancer was already tainting my first precious months with my daughter. How much longer was it set to go on for?

The operation was over but, now, the appointment with Mr Williams, where I was to discover the truth about my lymph glands, was looming. I felt that familiar fear kick in. Ash and I had made a pact to try not to talk about it – something that, given what he knew, must have been a huge relief to him.

There's always going to be a next hurdle, I thought, two days before my conclusive results were due, as I prepared Gigi's bottles. What if the cancer has spread to my lymph glands? This is only the beginning.

On Tuesday, just as another angry day loomed like a

raincloud, Gigi perked me up. I was always blowing bubbles at her and, that morning, she started blowing them back, dribbling all down her top.

'Clever girl!' I chirped in my proudest voice. It really made my day.

Instantly cheered, I put on my perfume, make-up and gladrags and took Gigi to meet some girlfriends for lunch. I needed to have some fun and feel carefree, to have a good old gossip and forget what was going on. Thankfully, my girlfriends totally delivered. In fact, my friends were proving to be incredible throughout all the stages of my illness so far.

One day, David, the husband of Tracey, one of my best friends, made an unbelievable offer. 'Please let me help you financially. If there's anything at all you need that will speed up the process, promise you'll let me know, so I can help,' he said.

He was prepared to pay for anything, which I thought was so touching. It was the same with Ash's dad, his uncle Russell, his aunt Ruth and his friend John, whose best man he'd been. These were offers I would never dream of taking them up on, but it was great to hear them at the time. I really did feel blessed that I was so loved.

One thing I could have done with some help with, though, were the piles of paperwork that went with having cancer. You wouldn't believe it. I kid you not, you need your own secretary to cope with the amount of forms there are to fill in and the information you need to read. Every test result, every appointment, all the private-healthcare forms and invoices, medication and treatment instructions, waivers and consents to show you'd had whatever step explained and that you had understood what was entailed . . . I now have a cheery 'cancer' folder on my desk at home dedicated to this time of my life. Honestly, it's an admin nightmare!

Nine days after the operation, Ash accompanied me back to the Spire for my results. Ash was gabbling away like a mad thing on the way there in the car, making very little sense, but I think it helped him get through the drive there, even if it did wind me up!

As we sat in the waiting room, I got talking to a very glamorous young mum who was with her little boy and her husband. She looked so amazing, I just assumed she was there to have a boob job or something. She was so happy and excited. I was chatting to her about Gigi, and she was asking me lots of questions about how I was finding motherhood and coping with the lack of sleep.

As lovely as she was, I couldn't help but think, Oh God, if I had a choice, I so wouldn't be here, volunteering for an operation. She probably thought I was there for cosmetic surgery too. It sounds silly, but I'd really glammed up that day, and was wearing a turquoise kaftan, and had big hair. It was as if putting on some kind of outside mask could protect me from the truth. I refuse to get bad news when

I'm looking and feeling like shit, I'd thought to myself that morning while blow-drying my barnet, channelling my inner Joan Collins.

After a short wait, Ash and I were called in to see Mr Williams.

He seemed pleased to see us, but I also got the sense that he had something serious to say.

'I need to look at your scar,' he said. 'Would you like me to tell you your results before or after I examine you?' he asked.

'Please tell me now,' I replied, as a real sense of foreboding kicked in.

'Well, the news is mixed,' he said. 'Basically, we did find tumour in your lymph glands. Nineteen out of thirty-three are affected.'

I felt as if I had been struck by a hammer. I was devastated. All the preparation for the operation, all the good food and positive thinking hadn't made a scrap of difference. I felt sick to my stomach, and my whole body was trembling.

'We need to book you in for a CT and a nuclear medicine bone scan,' Mr Williams continued. 'Then we'll know what we're faced with.'

I noticed Ash looking at me with a mix of sympathy and sorrow, and squeezing my hand. He looked gutted but not surprised at the news. Now, his dark mood during my recovery after the operation in hospital made sense. I tried to concentrate as Mr Williams carried on: 'So we need to book you in for those scans as soon as we can. In fact, we need to book you in right now. There's not a minute to lose.'

7. My Own Casualty

Standing over Gigi's cot, I studied my daughter sleeping peacefully, tucked up under a pink blanket. She looked so cute, with her mop of brown hair and squeezable little cheeks.

'I swear she's smuggling nuts in those cheeks,' Ash always joked. 'She's just like a little squirrel.'

He was right, and she looked adorable. For a moment, I envied her innocence and ability to sleep soundly, sure that all was right with the world.

No matter how bleak things got, Gigi was always the one thing that kept me going. From the moment I found out I had cancer, I made a vow to be strong around her.

It occurred to me that we become what our parents instill in us at an early age. I kept thinking of that famous saying, 'Give me the child until he is seven, and I will show you the man.' The first few years of a baby's life are so important, and I knew instantly that I couldn't let my illness blight the way I was with Gigi. She had her routine, and I needed to stay constant, focused and upbeat. I didn't want her to sense there was anything wrong.

I'm not going to do this miserably, I vowed to myself. If I have any 'moments', they won't be in front of her. If I can do my best to protect her from all of this, I will. But it wasn't going to be easy, that was for sure.

When I heard that nineteen out of my thirty-three lymph glands had been invaded by cancer, I immediately feared the worst: That the cancer had spread beyond control, my life was over and, most excruciating of all, that Gigi would grow up without her mother. I thought, Oh my dear Lord, I've had it. That's it. I'm done. It sounded as if my whole body was riddled with cancer. That it was busy consuming me, breaking me down with every minute that passed.

Whenever I've heard the words 'lymph glands' in relation to cancer, it's made me think about death. I was sure that, if cancer got into your lymphs, then you were a goner. After all, that meant it wasn't contained or confined – it was travelling around me, potentially settling in and taking up residence elsewhere. Now, it seemed like my worst fear was coming true.

Sitting in that office with Ash and Mr Williams, I found myself desperately searching for something positive to hang on to.

'Nineteen is just over half,' I told myself. 'He's not telling me they're all affected.' Then I realized that Mr Williams was still talking and that I had better listen. So I sat there, shell shocked, as he explained how the lymph glands are the body's filtering system.

'It could mean that your lymphs have done their job of filtering the cancer to stop it,' he said. 'But it could also mean that it's spread to other parts of your body. That's what we need to find out.'

Hearing the news, I swallowed hard. I could feel the panic rising up through my body. I felt sick – sick to the stomach, and petrified about the future. 'It could be OK,' I said to myself, over and over. 'I mean, they could still be going for total cure.'

The shock and despair must have been written all over my face, because Mr Williams was studying me with a real look of compassion.

'Rebekah, there's good news, too,' he said kindly. 'During the operation, I took a cut from the tissue around the tumour, and that has been tested. On the up side, we have a very clear surrounding area of tissue, so it hasn't spread in the immediate area. We just need to check that the cancer isn't anywhere else either.'

Up until then, I'd been holding my breath but, now, I allowed myself to exhale deeply. Well, that was something to hang on to.

'What happens with the scans?' asked Ash. He spoke calmly, but I knew him well enough to know he was struggling to keep it together.

What must he be going through right now? I wondered. Is he thinking what I'm thinking? That I might be dead this time next year?

Mr Williams explained that I needed to be staged (a medical term which means they work out what stage your body is at with the cancer), and this could be done with the bone scans, which they would analyse to see if they could spot the cancer anywhere else.

'After you've been staged, you'll start your chemo in the next few weeks,' he told me. 'The other good news is that tests have shown you're sensitive to Herceptin.'

I let out another big lungful of air. That was a very good thing. I knew Herceptin was an amazing drug, which had been proven to benefit women with my type of breast cancer. Trials had indicated that the risk of a tumour returning after surgery, radiotherapy and chemotherapy was halved when Herceptin was used for a year post-surgery, either with other drugs, or on its own. It was reassuring to know I was lining up the best defences against cancer. But, still, with everything else I'd heard that day, it seemed a little bit early to be whooping triumphantly or high-fiving Ash. Instead, I squeezed his hand and smiled.

'If she didn't have chemotherapy, radiotherapy and Herceptin, what would happen?' asked Ash nervously.

'We call this belt and braces,' replied Mr Williams. 'We can't tell you either way, but it's really good for you to have both the belt and the braces to offer you extra support and protection.'

Next, Mr Williams asked to examine the area of my lumpectomy to see how it was healing.

'Ooh, that's a wonderfully neat scar,' the nurse Maggie, who'd been sitting in, commented, admiring his handiwork.

'It's one of the best I've ever done,' he replied, smiling.

I smiled back, but it didn't bother me either way. All I could think about was the scans and what was to come, all the uncertainty that was still swirling around. The superficial stuff didn't matter to me.

'Someone will call you soon to arrange your appointments,' Mr Williams promised, as we got up to leave.

'Thanks,' I said, as graciously as I could. But, inside, I felt totally crushed.

When we walked out of the office, we were greeted by Dan, one of the hospital porters who'd looked after me while I was in hospital for my lumpectomy. He called us into a side room, along with Maggie, and told us to sit with her while he, sweetly, brought us tea and biscuits.

I'll tell you what, I needed that cup of tea. I was still reeling from the shock. You see, after recovering from the operation, I'd been hell bent on receiving some good news. I'd hardly allowed myself to think about anything else. But, yet again, I felt like I'd had a sledgehammer slammed down on me. The situation with my lymph glands guaranteed that there would be yet more unrest, more fear of the unknown, and more silent prayers as I was forced to wait for results.

Feeling restless and anxious, I sat there, fidgeting. I had to really concentrate on everything I said to Maggie, and I was struggling to get my words out coherently. My head was just so full of stuff. I felt all muddled, and Ash and I got angry for the first time. We couldn't believe it had spread, the reality was, this was just the beginning. Ash was wringing his hands so tightly his knuckles were white. He stood up so abruptly, the chair flew out behind him, went over to the wastepaper bin and gave it a really big kick, which sent it clattering over the other side of the room. I was mortified, but Maggie just took it all in her stride. She was such a kind woman, and offered us a really sympathetic ear. As Ash and I sat there bewildered, trying to get our heads round everything, she had this very calming way of nodding her head, which really pacified us.

We had a million questions, but we didn't know where to start. We didn't know where we were going and felt totally lost.

Of course, I'd known there was a possibility that the cancer had spread to my lymphs. That was why they'd taken a biopsy. But that didn't make it any easier. The fact that over half my lymph glands had tumour in them was a very bitter pill to have to swallow.

When we left the hospital, I went straight into 'operation cancer' mode, marching into the nearest healthfood shop to stock up on all the complementary medicines and extras I had been told might help: soya milk, enzyme tablets, bucketloads of vitamin C tablets, and green tea. I also bought lots of deodorant, without aluminium. I'd been told to avoid aluminium ones, as scientists were still questioning whether there was a link between antiperspirants and breast cancer. I bought them for all my girlfriends, my mum and Jen too. As soon as I got home, I carried on my spree by unplugging the microwave and putting it away under the stairs – I'd decided that all those electrical waves couldn't be good for you. Internet research had told me in no uncertain terms that the human body's most important defence was its immune system. It is there to act as a firewall against colds, coughs or diseases, and to fight against the cancer cells should the body develop them. I knew the most important thing I could do now was to keep as healthy as I could. If my immune system was fighting fit, I reasoned, that would be half the battle won.

But, despite all my fighting talk, as I wandered down the high street in Tunbridge Wells, I felt numb. It still didn't feel real, and I wondered how long it would be before I learned what was really in store for me.

As it happened, I only had to wait a few days for the scans – the first one would be on Wednesday, and the second one on the Thursday – but it still seemed like for ever.

Dad and his wife Angie came up that weekend, it was actually the first chance they'd had to meet Gigi given everything that had been going on. It provided us with a welcome distraction – I don't think Ash and I felt we could really show just how much pressure we were under. Instead, we did our best not to mope around, but there was so much tension between us about the impending scans. We couldn't think of anything else. It was like the biggest sword of Damocles hanging over everything. If Dad hadn't been there, we might have wallowed in our black hole for the entire weekend, sniping at each other and opting for those long silences so we could pretend it wasn't happening to us, so we could pretend it wasn't for real. As it was, we went out and about and tried to forget.

On Sunday, we spent the afternoon going for a walk in the sunshine with them and, later, for dinner, but the news about my lymphs was always there, tapping away at me, taunting me with the endless ways the scenario could unfold.

On the Monday morning, I forced myself to get on with all the usual chores, and tried to be upbeat and carefree around Gigi.

While changing her nappy that morning, I noticed that she was lifting her head to look around. Oh my God, she's getting so big now, I thought. The milestones were coming thick and fast. At that moment, I felt eaten up by rage. I felt so angry and robbed, that my little girl was changing every day before my eyes and this bastard cancer was taking that away from me, it was distracting me from my most important role, from the thing I had wanted more than anything, from the thing I had planned for so meticulously. My desire to be a mother had been so powerful, so overwhelming – and, now, I wasn't even being allowed to do it properly. I wasn't like every other mum, I had breast cancer. Wham! Everything, even the most basic things, felt totally out of my control.

That afternoon, I went to the Kent and Sussex hospital to meet my oncologist, who also happened to be my neighbour, Rema. There are certain appointments you never want to make, and one at a clinical oncology department is right up there in first place. As soon as I sat down in her office, Rema handed me a glass of water and we started to talk through the chemotherapy and its side effects. As I listened to her, I felt like I couldn't breathe.

Rema could see I was struggling, and put a reassuring hand on my arm. 'Do you need a minute?' she asked, concerned 'Do you want a cup of tea, Rebekah?'

I looked up with tears in my eyes, but forced a smile. 'No, I'm good. I need to know what's what, don't I? No point hiding from it.' Anyway, the night before I'd read the pink leaflet given to me by the breast cancer nurse. It was entitled 'Everything You Need to Know about Radiotherapy and Chemotherapy'.

My God, it made for shocking reading. Even the definition of the treatment made me want to scream:

Chemotherapy is a treatment with drugs which control or destroy cancer cells. It also stops the cancer from dividing, growing and spreading . . . In the broad sense, most chemotherapeutic drugs work by impairing *mitosis (cell division)*, effectively targeting *fast-dividing cells*. As these drugs cause damage to cells, they are termed cytotoxic. Some drugs cause cells to undergo *apoptosis* (so-called 'programmed cell death').

I'd managed to keep calm going through it on my own at home, but talking about it here, in hospital, made it feel so real. Rema gave me an encouraging pat and sat back as she carried on explaining what I could expect. I thought back to that leaflet and the endless list of possible side effects. Even if I didn't suffer from a quarter of them – bloody hell, just one sounded awful enough:

Hairloss, including eyelashes, eyebrows and thinning of other body hair
Sickness
Loss of appetite
Diarrhoea and constipation (the drug will affect the nerve supply to the bowel for a while. Some anti-sickness drugs and painkillers can make it worse)
Numbness in limbs (hands and feet)
Fatigue
Ulcers and mouth sores (some may become infected)
Taste alterations
Loss of appetite
Kidney problems

Weakening in nails (you may lose them)
Skin changes
Temporary reduction in bone-marrow function
Bruising and bleeding
Weakening of the heart muscle

The sodding list went on for ever. I was facing six high-dosage sessions of chemotherapy, each session separated by twenty-one days to allow my body time to re-group and settle down again before the next blast. When Rema had finished going through it all, I was given another load of leaflets containing contact numbers and helplines, and then I signed my life away, confirming that I understood all the risks. Oh happy days! My bulging 'cancer file' was all the evidence I needed to remind me that the horror was only just beginning.

I'm not really into hippy claptrap, but my friend Michelle had been hounding me for some time to go and see a spiritual healer in Chelmsford and, finally, I had relented.

When we arrived there, just off one of the main bypasses, I was bemused to see that he worked out of an odd Tardis-like building, kind of like one of those temporary classrooms. Inside, it was filled with all the new-age paraphernalia, shrines and thousands of messages from people all over the world. It was utterly fascinating and, weirdly, quite comforting. I've always been interested in fate and the idea that there is something else or 'other', and I would certainly always choose a complementary potion over harsh medication if the situation allowed. I was so careful when I was pregnant about what went into my body.

To be honest, going somewhere to talk about healing was just what I needed as I tried to process that hideously long list of side effects I could expect once my treatment began. Anything natural, spiritual and positive was more than welcome.

Oh, what the heck, I thought, and handed over my £20.

The healer was called Steve, and he was this odd-looking giant of a man – about six foot five – with long hair. He was wearing a long white shirt and acted very seriously. But, I had to admit, he had a real aura about him.

Straight away, he started making these bizarre circular motions beneath my chest, kind of in the middle of my ribs, as if he was digging invisible matter out of my body and chucking it away. Then he pressed his hands gently on top of my clothes around my breast and armpit. 'It's out of you, isn't it?' he said. 'It's gone.'

I nodded.

He carried on like that for a while, issuing lots of deep movements, like he was pulling all the badness out of me.

'You'll feel tired later,' he said, 'so get lots of rest.'

By the time Michelle and I had had lunch and driven back to Tunbridge Wells, I felt a lot less stressed, but I was so exhausted I could hardly keep my eyelids open.

I arrived home, where Jen was looking after Gigi, but I didn't even have the energy to cuddle my baby. As soon as I got through the front door, I had to go straight up to bed. I felt terrible that I wasn't spending time with my little girl but, as my head hit the pillow, I knew I wasn't fit for anything.

The next day, I felt rested, but still on edge.

That night, I went to bed early, shattered from nerves and still very scared. There was nothing in my mind apart from the impending scan so, despite my extreme exhaustion, I lay there, wide awake and terrified. I recalled the healer's words – 'It's out of you, isn't it?' – and tried to be positive. But I just couldn't get it all out of my head.

Some time later, I heard Ash's footsteps on the stairs. He crept into bed and, although I tried to pretend I was asleep, I clearly wasn't fooling him.

'You all right, babe?' he asked me, as we lay there in the pitch dark.

'Yep,' I replied in a small voice.

'Babe, you're not, are you? Come on. Talk to me,' he pleaded.

'I don't want to. It's nothing,' I said, not wanting to go into it. There's only so much he can take, I thought. I need to try to protect him from all this. He's suffering too.

But Ash was persistent and, eventually, I crumbled into a sobbing wreck.

'Please tell me it's going to be OK,' I cried, my whole

body shaking. 'I feel as if I'm on a train gathering momentum. I want to get off, but I can't.'

I was in a right state. Here I was curled up next to the man I loved, the man who had helped me create the perfect little family, and I was facing the fact that I might die and leave it all behind.

'Becks, listen to me,' Ash said, holding me really tightly. 'Have I ever been wrong about anything? I'm promising you: you're going to be absolutely fine.'

But I caught the wobble in his voice, and I realized that he was talking to himself as much as he was to me. For Christ's sake – apart from each other, what else did we have?

That night was one of my darkest times, but Ash was fabulous. He held me and stroked my forehead in a bid to help me relax and sleep. I drifted off in the end, but I'm sure he didn't, as he was as pale as a ghost the next morning.

That morning, before the scan, we went to the chemo clinic at the hospital to be briefed on my treatment. I think it was then it really hit me: I was sitting in a f***ing chemo clinic.

Beforehand, I was sitting in the corridor, and I got chatting to a woman in her seventies, who told me her husband was having chemo. I explained what I was doing there too.

'I'm a bit scared,' I admitted.

'You're going to be fine,' she told me, which instantly made my eyes well up.

'Sorry, I'm getting emotional,' I mumbled, and she touched my arm kindly, which made me sniff even more. Then she handed me a tissue.

Just as I was about to have a good old weep, I was called in to see one of the nurses, Ellen.

'Coming on to the ward for the first time can be a very emotional thing,' she explained, seeing my watery eyes. 'Most patients have a moment when it dawns on them that it is really happening.'

After that, we had a long chat and went over the side effect again but, for most of the time, all I could think about was the scan that was coming up next.

After being briefed, we went straight for the scan. Ash and I were shown into the silent waiting room. He and I sat there speechless, watching all these different people from all walks of life coming and going. Suddenly, the fear set in. I was overwhelmed by panic because, everywhere you looked, there were sick people. It doesn't matter how much you kid yourself: you are all in the same boat, you are all, potentially, going to die from it. Most people there had undergone an operation of some sort to cut out the bad stuff. There were bald people, people shuffling on sticks and frames, people with drains and catheters to help rid them of fluids and toxins. There were others at the start of their journey. It was in that waiting room that I realized that, whatever I did, I had no choice: I was part of their gang.

I had to drink a huge cup of a vile-looking orange

contrast before having the scan. It took me for ever to get it down. I gagged repeatedly, the residue sticking to my gums and lodging in the back of my throat. I noticed there were loads of other people in the waiting room, also knocking it back. All these patients, all with their own dramas going on. Then it was time for me to go in.

I was called by a man in his twenties, who was very kind and patient. He explained that the scan would give them a series of X-rays, which would help them to build up a picture of the inside of my body and see if there were any more tumours.

I lay down on a bed that was a bit like a conveyor belt, which manoeuvred me head first into the scanner. It was like a tiny tunnel. I wasn't sure how on earth I would fit into it. I felt utterly claustrophobic, my whole body trembling with apprehension.

I knew I was supposed to be lying there really still, but I couldn't help but move. The more I tried to concentrate on controlling my jerking limbs and keeping my breathing relaxed, the more I was twitching and moving, but the young man didn't get irritated with me.

'Try and stay still,' he said softly. He was really gentle and compassionate. He didn't have to be nice like that, but he was.

At every point of my cancer treatment I've been overwhelmed by how kindly I've been treated. All the women on reception, all the staff at the hospitals, they've been so sensitive to my feelings, and they've really taken the time to be sympathetic without being full of pity, without showing their own fear that it could happen to them at any time, without that cloying 'How *are* you?' When you are feeling frightened and low, being treated like that makes such a difference. We've got some really special people working in the NHS and private hospitals.

That night, I couldn't eat, I was so nervous about the results.

'Please try and have something,' Ash begged, but I couldn't. I just felt knotted up inside.

Because it had taken so long for me to be diagnosed properly, my biggest fear, right from day one, was that the cancer had spread. I couldn't bear the thought that it might have got me before I even had a chance to fight it. I needed hope, I needed to know that the outcome was within my control. I didn't want to face the impossible stuff, I just wanted to know that I had a chance of recovery.

On Thursday morning, after a restless night, I dropped Gigi off at Jen's house again as I was booked to have a mildly radioactive substance injected into my veins to show up any lurking cancer cells in my next bone scan. I had to avoid exposing Gigi to it, so we'd made plans for Jen to look after Gigi until the Saturday.

Charlotte came with me to the hospital, and we dashed in like Anneka Rice on a challenge, assuming we were late.

As it happens, we weren't and, as we sat, waiting, my

mobile rang. It was a withheld number, and my stomach lurched. Rema had said she would call as soon as she had my first set of results.

'Hello,' I answered tentatively. It *was* Rema.

'How are you?' she asked.

'Fine – what's the news?' I asked, keen to get to the nitty-gritty.

'Rebekah, I'm so pleased to tell you – your first scan has come back clear,' she said. 'So hopefully the next one will be fine too.'

Well, I nearly jumped for joy. Gabbling the news to Charlotte, I quickly called Ash.

'It's all good!' I babbled. 'The scan has come back clear!'

I could hear him whooping with joy and telling everyone at work. He was elated, so were all the boys.

When I went in for the injection, I was telling my good news to anyone who'd listen, to the extent that I'd almost forgotten I was going in to have needles stuck in me. I didn't much like injections – but now, frankly, it was the least of my problems. Once the nurse had finished using me as a pincushion, she told us we had three hours to kill before the scan.

So Charlotte and I hit the shops. We had our make-up done and went for lunch.

Back at the hospital, the bone scan was a breeze, now that so much of my fear had gone and afterwards I headed home, my spirits considerably raised.

Ash and I really wanted to celebrate that night but, after everything we'd been through, we thought we'd better err on the side of caution, so we called up our friends and asked them to meet us at our favourite Italian the following night.

Then we settled in for an evening at home, enjoying a lovely dinner and an early night. For the first time since Gigi's birth, it was just me and Ash, and it was a real treat to spend some quality time together. We tried to be upbeat about the good news we'd had – I liked to think it was a good omen and the start of a real positive path through this cancer maze, but I knew that, although Ash was humouring me, he was still feeling anxious. I can always tell what he is thinking. I also knew, however, that he was delighted to see me so upbeat. He wasn't going to let anything spoil it.

The following morning it was back to Carry on Cancer (as I was beginning to dub my never-ending schedule of injections, scans and appointments). This time, I was having an implant put into my stomach. I'd have to have this done every month, before the next blast of chemo.

It was part of a trial I'd signed up for in a bid to lower the chances of my treatment affecting my fertility. It had been odd making the decision to take part as, like all women my age suffering from cancer, I'd had to think long and hard about whether I wanted more children.

Rema had warned me that chemo attacks all fast-growing cells, so it could affect my ovaries, leaving me temporarily or permanently infertile. But, she revealed, if I chose to have this implant, Zoladex, it could help 'shut down' my ovaries and therefore protect them from the treatment. It would temporarily turn off the signals from the brain that tell your ovaries to make oestrogen – essential for my type of cancer, and for anyone with cancer thinking of having more babies.

Ash and I had discussed it long and hard.

If I was honest with myself, the thought of having more children really frightened me. It made me nervous that I'd developed a cancerous tumour while I was pregnant with Gigi. I couldn't help but wonder if my pregnancy hormones had somehow played a part in its development. Your body is so up in the air when you're pregnant, it's as if it's been invaded. If I'd got cancer once while I was expecting, surely it was plain stupid to attempt to get pregnant again and potentially open my body up to the same situation? I'd even got chatting to a girl in Costa Coffee, who told me her friend had got breast cancer after both her pregnancies. In the end, though both Ash and I felt blessed to have had one child, we decided it would be nice to have the option to have more children if we wanted. I didn't want the cancer to rob me of all my choices.

So, we'd eventually agreed to the implant, to bolster our chances. It didn't affect any aspect of my treatment, and we could always decide not to have children when the time came. Another factor that helped me make the decision was the hope that it might help guard me against early menopause – another side effect of chemotherapy. It was daft, but menopause, and all that went with it, terrified me – the hot flushes, the weight gain, everything. To me, it signalled the end of my youth, my childbearing years, my freedom of choice. Christ, my mum hadn't long gone through it!

After my injection that morning, I drove to the train station to meet Jane, my oldest friend, who was coming to visit from London. As I sat waiting in the car, a withheld number came up again. It was Rema. Thankfully, she skipped the niceties.

'I've got your bone scan results,' she said. 'You're all clear.'

Hanging up, I clutched the steering wheel with my hands and rested my forehead on it. I just felt so, so relieved. I finally felt I had a real chance of beating this thing.

When I met Jane I told her my good news and she engulfed me in a big hug. I don't think I've ever felt so happy.

That evening, Ash, Jane and I headed out to dinner with our friends, and I had a glass of champagne to celebrate.

I wanted to make the most of the joy I felt, but I knew I still had plenty more mountains to climb. Once again, just like when I was preparing to have Gigi, I was tackling my cancer like a job, like a mission to be accomplished. Pre-planning Prevents Poor Performance and all that!

In a pre-emptive strike, I'd arranged to go for regular sessions of acupuncture, to try to defend against any infection or low blood counts the chemo might cause. My first session was the following day. I was determined not to miss one lot of chemo, so I knew I had to be in tip-top condition. I wanted to crack on and get it out of the way.

But, just as before every stage I had already been through, a real sense of foreboding was setting in. And it wasn't even the treatment that bothered me – it was the thought of losing my hair.

A few days before my chemo began, I was brushing my long chestnut locks, and it really hit home that me and my beloved barnet were living on borrowed time. The thought filled me with horror and sadness. Every time I looked in the mirror, my bald head would be an instant reminder that I was ill. Every time I walked down the street, it would be an immediate sign to every stranger who saw me that I was sick, that I was a cancer victim. And I didn't want to be reminded of that. I didn't want people making that connection, lowering their eyes and trying not to look at the 'woman with cancer'. I didn't want anyone's pity, least of all my own.

'Stop it, Rebekah,' I told myself sternly, staring at my reflection in the mirror. 'You're not losing your eyesight or any limbs. Your hair will grow back! How can you be this vain? Get a grip. It's about living, that's all. It's about surviving.'

But losing my hair still seemed like the worst imaginable side effect. I'd had long hair for the last fifteen years. I couldn't bear the thought of it coming out in long clumps, of losing some of it and having thin, limp strands left. I didn't want my long, glossy-looking mane to look dull and patchy. All the magazines say you can tell so much by the state of someone's skin and hair. I didn't want to *look* ill any more than I wanted to *be* ill.

A few days earlier, I'd chatted to my friend Michelle about my fears.

'I've decided I want to get it cut in preparation,' I'd told her.

She explained that she'd heard about a service the celebrity hairdresser Trevor Sorbie had set up to help women with medical hair loss to adjust to the situation.

'He helps you choose the right wig, and then he cuts it to suit you,' Michelle enthused.

She called him up for me and he kindly fitted me in for a consultation on the Tuesday before my chemo began.

When I met Trevor, he was just amazing. He told me that his sister-in-law had been through cancer and, when she'd confided about the terrible feelings of unattractiveness she'd been forced to face up to, it had inspired him to help others in the same situation.

'I want every town in the country to have this service,' he said. 'I'm going to devote the rest of my career to it.'

While he was helping me to pick out a wig, he

introduced me to a sweet six-year-old girl who had leukaemia and had come over from Germany for his help. I immediately felt like there was a reason why we had met. I couldn't even begin to imagine what she was going through and felt quite ashamed of all the moaning I'd been doing and how full of self-pity I'd been of late. 'Get over it, Beck!' I said to myself, irritated at how pathetic I'd been.

I arranged to go back the following day to have my hair cropped into a nice, sharp bob. But, as positive as I tried to be that morning, I couldn't go back to sleep after Gigi's 4 a.m. feed. There were no two ways about it – I didn't want to lose my hair. The cancer is life-threatening – why on earth am I so concerned about my appearance? I chastised myself, but I wasn't feeling much better by the time I got to the salon.

After I'd had my hair washed and prepped, I sat in the chair staring at my reflection.

'OK, Rebekah?' Trevor said, appearing behind me.

'Yes,' I lied, very unconvincingly.

As Trevor began to chop away, I bit my lip and let my mind wander back to my *Casualty* days. There was one storyline in which Nina's half-sister Ellen had cancer and Nina had helped to cut her hair in preparation for her cancer treatment. During the scene, Nina had hacked off great big chunks of Ellen's hair, sobbing uncontrollably as she did so. It all seemed a bit OTT now.

Being pampered helped to make my experience more

exciting than sad, but it was odd none the less. There were loads of glossy fashion magazines, endless tea, coffee, juices and cakes. It was first-class treatment, that's for sure.

When Trevor had finished, I studied my reflection. I didn't really know what to make of it. It was weird having such short hair. My head felt lighter, for one thing.

I wonder if Gigi will recognize me, I thought. Then I felt guilty. Why had I let worries about my hair stop me spending time with my daughter for the last two days? Why hadn't I been concentrating on her needs? I couldn't wait to get home to her. I flicked my new bob all the way back to Tunbridge Wells on the train.

When I got home, Gigi acted as if nothing was up – I got the usual gummy smile from her as she cooed and blew bubbles. To her, I was just Mummy, and that was the biggest relief. Ash loved my new haircut too, he reckoned it made me look very smart and sophisticated – and younger. Bless him, he tried to convince me that he preferred it to how I had had it before, even though I knew my hair was one of the things he loved most about me – but hey, who was I to argue? It was just what I wanted to hear.

As I put Gigi to bed that night, I felt a new resolve wash over me – I was ready to take this bastard illness on. I had taken one small step in the right direction – and my haircut became a symbol of hope, of me taking back a bit of control and psyching myself up for what lay ahead. I was ready to face it, come what may.

8. *The Harsh Reality*

The morning of my chemo, I woke up feeling strangely calm.

I've bought the ticket for the show, now let's get it over with, I thought, as I arrived at the hospital with Ash.

On the ward, we were welcomed by a team of four nurses.

I noticed one of them was looking at me, a bit of a bemused look on her face.

'Sorry to ask this,' she said. 'We heard a rumour that you used to be on *Casualty*?'

It was a welcome distraction. Suddenly, I wanted to live up to Nina's feisty, hardcore reputation, the plucky paramedic, always strong and never scared. So I put on a brave face. But, as they prepped me up, with a tube going into my right wrist, and administered a dose of anti-sickness drugs, I caught sight of the bright, neon-pink tube of drugs waiting to be pumped inside me.

This was it. I was here, with a drip in my right arm, watching chemo go into my body. It didn't get any scarier than this.

My eyes welled up, and I felt all panicky. I don't want that toxic crap in my veins, I thought. I should be playing with my baby, taking her for long walks in her pram and enjoying her, not watching poison drip into my body.

I also wondered what would happen if they got the dosage wrong? I had heard it could cause damage to your heart. In fact, it was at times like this, mulling over the endless side effects and possibilities, that I wished I hadn't read so much cancer literature after all. But I was also aware that this marked the moment that I would lose my hair. Everything was changing against my will, and I felt unbelievably sad and utterly furious. I just didn't want to be here, confronting the bad news, acknowledging that this disease had invaded my body. Living out my fear.

Seeing that I was having a wobble, Ash squeezed my hand tight and, comforted, I swallowed hard and tried my best to find my courage again.

I don't know how I really expected the chemo to feel but, after all my fears, it wasn't particularly dramatic. There was a funny taste in my mouth and a tingling round my eyes, but I didn't feel sick.

Two hours passed, and I just sat there, trying not to think about it. Instead, I laughed and joked around with Ash until, finally, I was released.

'How's my hair looking?' I laughed as we got in the lift. But I was only half-joking. I'd been given the option of wearing an ice cap for each chemo session. The idea behind it was that it kept the head and scalp really cool, which helped to minimize the hair loss while the toxic chemo pumped and pulsed its way round the body. I had already been told before the session that, because my cancer was so aggressive, the chemo I was having was mega strong. That meant the ice cap would have little effect and was unlikely to save my tresses, so I decided not to bother wearing it.

In all honesty, it was so heavy, and it felt like just one more thing to be endured, only to be disappointed when my hair fell out anyway. And I didn't need any more disappointments, however small.

When I got back home, I started to feel a bit weird. It was a toxic feeling – heavy and tired and bloated – so I went to bed. By early evening, I was hit by a juggernaut of sickness.

It came out of nowhere, a completely violent nausea. I had to hold on to the wall to try to balance myself. After that, I was sick once more, and I crawled into bed, the daunting reality that I'd have to go through this five more times hitting me. I was petrified, and it is no exaggeration to say I felt like I was dying. It was totally uncontrollable, and I hated it.

I curled up into a ball. I didn't even have the energy to cry. I don't want this, and I just can't do it, I thought. I'm not strong enough, I thought.

The following morning, I woke up feeling clammy and sick. So, for once, I gave in where Gigi was concerned, and

Ash played Mum, popping out to do some shopping with her while I dozed.

They came back armed with goodies like fruit and bread, but I still felt vile and I couldn't get out of bed, let alone face eating anything. Now I knew why everyone having chemo on that ward looked so thin – even the thought of food made me want to be sick all over again. Desperate for some relief, I called my acupuncturist from bed.

'Can you make the sick feeling go away?' I asked.

Later, I forced myself to get up and go to see him. At his premises, I lay there, feeling as if I was going to die as he put needles into my right wrist for sickness and into my shins for immunity. Magically, the waves of nausea started to subside.

However, over the next few days, I continued to feel chemically hungover, so I was relieved when Mum arrived from Devon to look after me for a few days. Somehow, just having your mum near is so comforting.

After the violent nausea, it was the tiredness that knocked me for six.

I needed injections every day, which artificially boost your immunity, and Ash bravely offered to administer them. I dubbed him Dr Ash, which he looked chuffed about. I think he was delighted to be able to do something to help.

The days started to fly by, in a haze of appointments. It never stopped: acupuncture twice a week, daily injections for immunity, my oncologist appointment on a Monday before chemo, which was every third Friday of the month, Zoladex injections just before every chemo session, tests before chemo to check my bloodcount. It was exhausting and meant yet more time away from Gigi, missing out on more moments I would never get back. It felt as if about a year had passed (in reality it was just a month) since the operation.

Then, around ten days after my first chemo session, I noticed that my hair was starting to thin but was yet to fall out. Some days, I'd almost be too scared to check it, others I'd be literally pawing it in front of the mirror twenty times a day.

'In a way I'll be glad when it does finally happen,' I told Ash. One positive thing at that time was that, now that my scar was pretty much healed, Mr Williams had permitted me to start swimming again. Stepping into the water felt amazing. As I did my first lap, I thought to myself, This'll heal me, and with each length, I felt stronger and stronger.

Two weeks and a day after my first chemo session, I woke to find piles of hair on my pillow. Although I'd been expecting it, it was still incredibly shocking. I spent the morning walking round gingerly, hardly daring to run my fingers through my hair in case any more fell out.

After a while, though, I decided enough was enough. Why should I be all miserable, watching it coming out in clumps, I reasoned with myself. So I skipped the shower that day and called my hairdresser, who promised to come round as soon as she could.

Jo was a sweet girl. She'd been cutting my hair for a while, and we'd become quite friendly. She'd never been to my house before, and I was amazed by the way she just took charge.

'This is what we're going to do,' she announced. 'This is a product for your scalp and, afterwards, we're going to give you a really lovely grade four, choppy choppy choppy . . .'

She just talked me through it all. 'Now let's put some music on and I'll give you a head massage,' she suggested brightly.

She was amazing.

Ash gave us each a glass of champagne in a bid to re-create the luxurious Trevor Sorbie experience, and then Jo set to work with her clippers, trimming my hair to a grade four. It cheered me up to see Gigi sat in her pyjamas in her little recliner, looking on wide-eyed and very amused.

Now I was actually doing something proactive, I felt quite calm. It did make me think back to that horrible scene on *Casualty* again, though.

I recalled that the producers had been keen to focus on the vanity, and the physical side of things, and they'd made a really big deal of chopping off Ellen's hair. Although we researched it well, it made me cringe thinking back to what a big deal I'd thought it was at the time. We rehearsed it a lot but, obviously, had only one take in which the character's hair was actually cut. I didn't want to do it – the actress, my friend Georgina, had waist-length blond hair, for God's sake. But there I was, doing the big crying scene, while I hacked off another girl's hair. It wasn't real life, it was just another acting scene for my showreel. It was only now, as life was imitating art, that I truly understood all the emotions that were tied up in losing your hair to chemo. It was soul-destroying.

'But it's the least of your worries, babe,' Ash kept saying, but it didn't make it any easier.

As it happens, a few weeks later I didn't give two hoots that I was as bald as Kojak but, at that particular moment, I was struggling to accept that my physical appearance was changing. I knew I was going to look ill and that people would immediately associate the way I looked with cancer.

Once Jo had finished my hair, I felt calmer, but I'd be lying if I didn't admit I was gutted too. It was really painful to see my hair in such a short, boyish crop. I didn't think it suited me at all – not that I had long to worry about that. Two days later, Jo was back with her clippers and, this time, I ended up looking like GI Jane (although not quite as gorge as Demi, sadly).

In those forty-eight hours, I'd been moulting all over the place – on my pillows, over Gigi's blankets, in her cot. Frustrated and upset, I tied a scarf over my hair and tried to distract myself by pruning my little girl. But, as I set to work filing down Gigi's nails so she didn't scratch her face, I paused to look up and saw she was staring at me. She looked like a wise old owl. I kissed her on the nose, and she reached up and stroked my scarf.

That moment of tenderness floored me. I sobbed my heart out. It reminded me once again that I was fighting this for Gigi, for Ash. For our family unit.

Weirdly, after fixating on it for so long, when Jo shaved my hair off completely, I felt immense relief. I was free of all the anxiety the thought of my hair loss had caused. I decided that I wasn't going to get upset any more, I was just going to remember that losing my hair meant that the chemo was working.

My biggest fear that day was that Ash would no longer find this incarnation attractive but, when he saw me, he couldn't have been any sweeter.

'You look beautiful, babe,' he said, looking at me fondly and rubbing my head tenderly. 'I fancy you more than ever.' He winked at me. Blimey, who'd have ever thought he'd dig the Sinead O'Connor look!

After a day or two, I actually felt quite proud of my bald head. I decided that I wanted to do something to mark what had happened, so I asked Michelle's boyfriend, James, who is a great photographer and friend, to come round and take some pictures of me.

I spent ages putting my make-up on, and then I posed in my bedroom. I felt very glamorous, if you can believe it and, when I got the shots back, I was thrilled. It just goes to show that losing your hair doesn't make you ugly. It was actually quite empowering.

It was still a bit strange going out in public for the first time. My first outing was to the cinema with friends to watch *Sex and the City*. I was so scared; it felt like such a big deal.

We met for a pre-show dinner and, although I'd covered my head with a fuchsia scarf, I still felt like I was hit by a sea of stares as I walked into the restaurant. I felt so self-conscious that it was all I could do not to burst into tears.

It was like those first few days after Gigi was born. I was scared to go out because it was all so overwhelming. I wanted to run back to the car and hide, but then my friends got up one by one from the table they were sitting at and gave me a hug. My appearance didn't remotely faze them.

'You look great,' they trilled. 'You look gorgeous!'

I wanted to cry.

Later, I saw another bald lady, walking around, proud as Punch. She had a little girl with her, and she was just getting on with it. I admired the way she didn't appear to give a stuff.

A few days later, my second dose of chemo came round. It wasn't nearly as daunting as I thought it would be. After I had told her about my violent nausea, Rema had upped my dose of anti-sickness tablets, and I had all the vomit-avoiding tools people had recommended to me – things like motion-sickness bands and ginger tea.

This time, Mum came with me, and she was a very welcome calming influence. Nothing seems to faze my mum, and I love her for that.

I was wearing my honey-blond wig (I was trying to channel Jennifer Aniston, but I think perhaps it was more Rod Stewart) and, after the treatment, Mum took me for afternoon tea and cake. I'd assumed that the anti-sickness drugs would stop any nausea but, all of a sudden, it hit me again.

'I've got to get home,' I told Mum. It was like a fog creeping in. That all-too-familiar hot, clammy feeling of sickness itching back into my body. And when I was sick, it was just as violent and uncontrollable as last time. I felt possessed.

We grabbed the baby from Jen's, got back to the house, and I crawled into bed with the blinds shut. I slept with a sick bowl by my side throughout, as it could catch you when you least expected it.

Of course, Gigi, the little minx, who'd been really good all week, chose that night not to sleep through. As I struggled out of bed at 4 a.m., Ash tried to stop me.

'Rebekah, let me do it,' he urged, but I was having none of it, even though getting up in the night after chemo was ridiculously hard work.

'Not even chemo can stop a control freak,' I mumbled. I

had my own system with the bottles and feeding, and that was that!

After that second lot of chemo, I felt really low – for the first three days I felt sick then, for five days, I had no energy at all.

'Staying positive is so tough when I feel so tired and crap,' I confided tearfully to Michelle on the phone. 'I just want to curl up in a little ball and die.'

In a few days, however, I was feeling emotionally stronger.

'I know you're feeling better,' Ash remarked. 'I'm getting it in the neck again.'

It was true: we were back rowing and bantering and, later, I apologized for being unreasonable.

'I don't retaliate because you're poorly,' he joked. 'But, don't worry, once you're better, you won't get away with a thing.'

At the start of June, Gigi was weighed by our NHS midwife.

'She weighs one whole stone!' I told Mum on the phone afterwards. 'It only seems like yesterday she was seven pounds five! I'm so proud! I took lots of photos of her on the scales!'

Mum laughed, but she sounded a bit choked when she spoke:

'You sound just like your old self, Rebekah. You're sounding like you.'

She was right. For a little while, I'd lost my silly streak

and my ability to treat every little thing as an adventure, as something to celebrate. It felt great to get it back.

While I'd been going through my dramas, Madeleine had been having her own, as she underwent radiotherapy. And, at the end of June, we went out for dinner to mark the end of her treatment.

I took along a bottle of pink champagne. It was a real milestone for both of us. Even though we were both on different journeys, and at different stages, it was nice to be able to relate to each other on a general level. It's strange to think that I had a really close friend going through the same thing as me – it scared me to think how close to home this hideous disease was.

But you need that support network of other people going through the same thing. For instance, all through my chemo, I'd phoned my friend's mum, Carol, who'd had cancer. Sometimes, you just need to talk to people who've been there. I know there are people who don't like talking about it, who see illness as a weakness. I guess I was lucky that I could talk it through – not even cancer could render *me* lost for words!

Meanwhile, normal life had resumed in the Pitman/ Gibbs household. Another row with Ashley (his fault, naturally!) and a lot of grovelling resulted in the most amazing surprise – a gorgeous pram for Gigi.

It was ridiculously shallow, I know, but I'd been harping

on about a new pram for ages, and Ash couldn't resist telling me he'd ordered one for Gigi from our favourite baby shop. The news made me jump for joy. It's funny how the smallest things can lift you in the middle of the most intense moments. The pram was pure decadence and, when it arrived, complete with a big pink bow, I nearly deafened Ash with my high-pitched squeal of delight.

'Gigi and I will get all dressed up and go for a promenade!' I announced grandly, while he shook his head, laughing.

However, although my sense of humour had returned, I still had my moments.

'If I have to tell one more person I have breast cancer, I'm going to scream,' I ranted to Mum one day.

It had been happening a fair bit. I'd be out and about, and an old friend would spot me. It sounds awful but, when I saw them approaching, it would fill me with dread. Although I found it therapeutic chatting things through with close friends, there were times I just wanted to ignore the fact that I had cancer, just to be normal, especially with people who weren't really close friends. Admitting it to people I hadn't seen for a while almost felt like admitting failure. It simply wasn't part of the 'where will we all be in ten years' plan. I didn't want the pity, and I certainly didn't need reminding how grim it all was.

By now, I'd ditched my Jennifer wig. It was tight around my head, a bit restricting, and it just felt fake, so I'd resorted to wearing headscarves instead.

When my friends clocked me, it didn't take a rocket scientist to work out I was in the midst of chemotherapy. While I appreciated people's sympathy and concern, reciting my tale of woe repeatedly brought on a wave of sadness. It made me sink into it.

'I don't want to go over it again and again,' I whinged to Mum. 'It's hard not to be rude but, sometimes, I don't want to talk about it.'

That was why I liked meeting up with the girls from my NCT group. There were eighteen of us, all with babies of a similar age, and we'd chat about our little darlings, work and life in general – but never about the Big C, thank the Lord. With them, I could just be a new mum, like them, instead of Rebekah cancer Gibbs.

In the afternoons, I'd taken to turning my phone off and sitting in the back garden with Gigi, reading a book while Gigi cooed contentedly, mesmerized by the windchimes. It was our little haven.

While I was gearing up psychologically for chemo session three, I also continued to swim regularly. It helped me to feel fitter and mentally stronger. In fact, I started to get into a weird treatment rhythm. It's scary how quickly even the most hideous of situations can become vaguely run of the mill.

'I feel strangely normal,' I told Rema.

'That's because your body excretes the drug very

quickly,' she explained. 'So, by the third week, your energy has come back.'

It was funny, because the fear I'd originally felt during my first chemo session had now been replaced by quite a jovial feeling of familiarity. Chemo became a little routine that I built into my day. Thankfully, my fitness levels before the treatment enabled me to get back on my feet quickly after each round.

When we arrived at the hospital for the third session, Ash presented the nurses with some chocolates. They quickly hooked me up. A couple of hours later, I was out the hospital like a shot and back home to bed.

'I've given in,' I told Ash as he brought me a cup of tea. 'I need rest, and I'm not going to fight it.'

'Good,' he said, kissing my forehead. 'Now make sure you do rest.'

Predictably, as the evening set in, the sickness crept up on me, and I vomited three times before collapsing back to sleep. My hands were also tingling, and I was terrified I would lose the feeling in them. How on earth would I cope, not being able to pick up my baby?

The next day, I felt really fragile, so Ash insisted on driving me to my acupuncture appointment. What has happened to my independence? I wondered. Feeling needy used to be something totally alien to me.

The tiredness continued on and off all that week, so I tried to sleep whenever Gigi did. Mum had arrived for the weekend of the chemo and immediately started fussing over us all.

We took a trip to the seaside that Sunday. Walking along the seafront wall in Eastbourne, I inhaled deeply, enjoying getting some fresh air into my lungs. Halfway there, I thought. Only three more sessions to go.

Back at home that evening, I even felt a glimmer of an appetite. Ash cooked a pasta dinner, but kept clowning around and creeping up behind me to inspect my head.

'You're still losing it!' he grinned each time.

'Get off!' I yelled, but it made me smile. We both knew that a bald head signalled that the chemo was working.

By now, Gigi had turned five months old and would sit angelically in her bouncy chair trying to join in with whatever was going on. She'd make this funny yelping noise, a kind of jubilant cry, which would be followed with a lovely smile when you turned to her.

She was developing her own little characteristics every day – learning how to blow bigger bubbles, rolling on her front and pointing her chubby fingers at everything and gabbling baby speak.

It was gorgeous. I'd just started her on solids, a big milestone. We liquidized some sweet potato and placed it carefully in her mouth with a little pink spoon. Her face was a picture! She just gazed at me in utter shock, before opening her mouth for more.

'I think she's going to be a real foodie,' I told Ash.

At moments like that, I hated the fact I was wishing my life with Gigi away, ticking off chemo sessions.

Another week brought another challenge – a mammogram to see if there were more tumours in my breasts and also to get a good 'file' picture of my post-op breasts, which they could use as a comparison for future check-ups. That was the thing about having cancer. You never had a chance to relax for long; there was always a new thing to worry about just around the corner, always something else to fear.

When I'd first been diagnosed in April, I was still breastfeeding, which made a mammogram impossible, so I'd had to hang on until my boobs were back to normal and the surgical scar had healed. I'd put the appointment off a few times but, now, I had finally made it in.

This time, having the X-ray taken was a quick and painless procedure. It consisted of ten minutes in front of a machine and, hey presto, I was on my way home, trying desperately to keep my mind off the worst possible scenario – that I would have more tumours. The irony didn't escape me that mid to late-thirties is when some women start thinking about going for a mammogram, and here I was having my first official one, already having had breast cancer.

'What if there's another lump lurking?' I asked Ash.

As usual, his answer soothed me, even if he did look terrified at the thought as he tried to calm me. Even so, all weekend, I felt haunted. Had it all been for nothing? All the hideous treatment, the hard work and positivity? What if the cancer was busy weaving its dark magic in other areas?

But, lo and behold, Monday afternoon brought the fantastic news we'd both been praying for. The mammogram had detected no more tumours.

Now, it was July, and I was counting down the days until 22 August – the date of my final chemo session.

'I'm thinking about organizing Gigi's christening,' I said to Ash as we cuddled up on the sofa. 'I think it'll be a good distraction.'

'That's good, babe,' he replied, switching the television over to watch *Match of the Day*.

'I'm thinking we could have it on her first birthday. By then, I'll hopefully be on the mend. We can invite all our friends and have a celebration,' I said.

'Yeah, sounds good,' he replied, eyes not wavering for a second from the football.

'And I thought Gary Lineker could be her godfather?' I tested.

'Sure. Whatever you want,' he answered, as I raised my eyebrows. Things were getting back to normal then!

That week, I asked Tracey, Amber and Michelle to be godmothers. They're all so dear to me and already such a huge part of Gigi's life. In her first six months, when I was desperate and distracted, they showed how much they loved her. I know they will teach her all the important things, if I'm not here to do it. If the unthinkable happens, and I'm not around in years to come, they'll tell Gigi all about what her mummy was like from a girlie perspective, I thought. They'll paint a lovely picture of all the fun we had together, singing and dancing. Of how much I enjoyed our time, made the most of it and fought to hang on to it.

At this point, Gigi's collection of girlie goodies was growing by the day. I almost hyperventilated with excitement when a pair of sparkly pink cowboy boots came from my cousin in Kansas. They were the campest thing I'd ever seen – but just brilliant.

When it came to chemo session number four, Rema explained that the remaining three courses were a different sort to the first three, so I wouldn't get the sickness side effect but a feeling of achiness instead. Like the worst flu you could ever imagine – and then some.

Well, the worst mistake I ever made was assuming it would be a walk in the park. Talk about tempting fate!

What I hadn't bargained for was a nasty reaction to the anti-sickness drugs I was taking, which led to my very own casualty drama.

Within twenty-four hours, something odd had started to happen. When I was feeding Gigi, Mum noticed that my tongue was extended out of my mouth and I was gurning, my jaw having gone numb. I didn't notice at first, but then I got a weird trembling feeling and my whole body began to shake uncontrollably.

Panicking, we rang the chemo helpline, who listened to my symptoms and insisted we call an ambulance, as they were worried I'd had some kind of stroke. Ash then called Rema, who told us it was probably a side effect, one a small number of women get from the anti-sickness drugs. Trust me to be one of them!

We called the ambulance for me, and Ash followed in the car, leaving Gigi at home with my mum.

I played Nina in *Casualty* for two years but, when we arrived at the hospital, I got my first real insight into the full-blown chaos A&E staff face every weekend. It was four hours before they were able to locate the right drug for me, and all we could do was sit silently as Saturday-night drunks shouted and hollered around us.

I couldn't speak. I felt really turned in on myself, like I was trapped in a bad dream. A lump formed in my throat and my bottom lip began to wobble. I can't cope with this, I thought. What the hell am I doing here on a Saturday night when I should be tucking up my baby and treating myself to a takeaway, like normal people? I don't want this alien taking over my life. I didn't ask for it, and I can't have it staying. I was exhausted. I needed this to be over. Thankfully, Ash spotted I was about to lose it. 'Don't do it, babe,' he soothed. 'Not here.'

Once I was seen, the doctors confirmed I'd had a reaction to the Metoclopramide (an anti-sickness drug) that I'd just started taking. Thankfully, after a delay, by 11.30 p.m., I'd had the injection I needed, my symptoms subsided, and I was allowed to head home.

Mum welcomed us back with fried-egg sandwiches. She said Gigi had been restless, almost as if she'd sensed something was up. Ash and I had hardly spoken on the way back. We were flagging under the pressure of being upbeat, boosting each other; we had run out of energy. Ash skipped his sandwich in favour of bed, desperate to sleep his mood away, and I wasn't long behind him, glad to see the back of the day.

I awoke to daylight pouring through the curtain on Sunday morning. I breathed a sigh of relief. I felt human again, so much so, I mistakenly sent my mum home. But, then, slowly, every bone in my body began to ache. On Monday, I could hardly drag myself out of bed. And the next few days, it was much the same.

Every time I got up to try and feed or bathe Gigi, I felt like I was going to faint, so I had to ask Ash's mum to look after her while he was at work.

'I feel as though I'm failing her as a mother,' I sobbed on the phone to Michelle. 'Now I understand why some people choose not to have chemo. It's awful. Until you've had it, you have no idea.'

I couldn't even pick up my own bloody daughter when

she cried – what kind of mother was I? I decided there and then that, even if the cancer came back, I was never going through chemo again.

The following day, I continued to feel sorry for myself. Ash came home and found me in bed watching an old comedy film. I could hardly crack a smile – until he sat next to me and started laughing. Before I knew it, I was doubled up, giggling with him.

Four days later, it was the Cancer Research UK Race for Life in Regent's Park. I'd been asked to take part, but I'd been so ill that I wasn't sure I'd be up to it. I knew that, as far as my awful reaction to the anti-sickness drugs was concerned, there was a danger zone my body temperature couldn't go into. If it did, I would have to go straight to hospital and be hooked up to a drip. I kept taking my temperature all the way there in the back of the car, worried that I wouldn't be well enough to take part, but when I got to Regent's Park and saw everyone so fired up, their enthusiasm was completely contagious. Ash had been so worried about me – in fact, he'd been nagging non-stop about how I wasn't well enough and that I was overdoing it. To be honest, it was all starting to get on my nerves, all these limitations cancer brought with it. I was sick of it. Sick of feeling like I couldn't, like I shouldn't. I just wanted my life back.

Before the race began, I was asked to go on stage and say a few words to the crowd. But what do you say to five thousand people, who all have their own stories about how cancer has affected their lives?

I took Gigi up with me, in the hope she'd help me find some words of encouragement. Her little face was a picture as she looked out at the sea of people, and I suddenly felt really choked. There was an eerie silence. I could really feel the audience's empathy.

'Thank you so much for coming. You are all amazing,' I managed to splutter. 'What a wonderful charity this is.' The words were getting caught in my throat, so I kept it brief.

Then I got to hoot the horn to start the race! I'd always wanted to do that!

I set off walking, and Ash pushed Gigi in her pram. She even had her own little entry number stuck on it with her name printed on it. She was officially the youngest participant in the race.

I finished the 5km walk feeling completely exhilarated but, on our way home, I realized my temperature had gone up to 38°C – which is in the danger zone if you're having chemo. I called the chemo helpline, and they instructed me to get straight to the hospital. For the second time in a week, I was back in A&E for a blood test. There was a possibility that I was neutropenic, a condition in which the blood is unable to fight infection. It can be a disaster for those undergoing chemotherapy and can lead to you being admitted to hospital for up to five days, kept in an isolation ward and put on a drip for antibiotics.

The doctors warned me that, if my temperature got any higher, I would need to be admitted but, luckily, it subsided again and, after the doctors had monitored me for a while, I was given the all clear and told to go home and rest. Thankfully, Jen and Rod were on hand to take charge of Gigi until I felt better.

A week later, I was washing my face when I noticed something really exciting – tiny little tufts of hair beginning to sprout out of my Kojak slaphead!

'Ash!' I yelled. 'Look! My hair is growing back!'

'Shame,' he said, stroking my head. 'I much prefer you as a baldy!'

Just like the previous session, my penultimate course of chemo would not be without drama.

The session started as normal, with me getting wired up and chatting away to the nurse but, after about two minutes or so, I suddenly felt really hot and flushed. I could feel the chemicals pumping through my veins, and my chest started to feel constricted, like someone was crushing me.

Jo, the nurse, took one look at my bright-red face and switched off the machine. My heart was racing, and my blood pressure was up. I was obviously having a reaction to the treatment.

A consultant was called, and Mum comforted me, as I bit my bottom lip and tried not to cry.

'I'm not worried about the reaction,' I confided in a trembling voice. 'I just don't want any hold-ups or delays.'

'Take it easy and calm down. Try not to upset yourself,' she told me. 'You'll just have to see what happens.'

But, for me, there was no room for manoeuvre – 22 August was the start of my new, chemo-free life, and I couldn't bear the thought of it being snatched away from me and dragged out for months more. I felt I just couldn't do it for a minute longer.

After two hours, during which I was treated with an anti-inflammatory steroid and antihistamines, I was relieved to be given the all clear to try again.

At first, I didn't even realize that Jo had turned the machine back on, I was so busy chatting away. She'd craftily started it up on the sly so that I wouldn't feel panicked. This time, I had no reaction against it and, when the treatment was complete, I walked out of there feeling brilliant.

As soon as I got home, I shouted, 'I'm now on the home stretch.' I grinned at Ash. 'It's nearly bloody over!'

Of course, within a few days, the aches were back. Just standing up to blend Gigi's lunch of pear and sweet potato made me feel as if I'd performed a matinee of *Starlight Express* with flu.

Thankfully, I'd found a way to amuse her which involved very little effort on my part. We'd recently treated her to a pink baby bouncer, which we suspended from the door frame. The minute I put her in it, she loved it. Her little legs were flailing as she bounced her up and down, giggling.

Ash found me in the front room, creased up with laughter. 'It looks like your dancing!' I guffawed. Ash does this kind of comedy eighties thing on the dance floor, and Gigi was doing the same!

'I don't know what you're on about,' he huffed, but I could see he was struggling not to laugh too.

Two weeks before my final stint of chemo, Madeleine made everything all the more poignant by sending me something really thoughtful in the post. It was a page from one of those calendars where you tear off a new date every day to find an inspiring message.

The page she sent me featured a quote from the French essayist Michel de Montaigne. It read: 'The value of life lies not in the length of days but in the use we make of them.' And the date? 22 August, of course! It totally summed up the way I felt about life at that moment.

Feeling better, I decided to accompany Ash to a classic cars fair near our home. There were hundreds of things I'd rather have been doing and, usually, I'd cry off but, instead, I smiled and tried to feign enthusiasm.

We put Gigi in her pram and met Amber, his aunt, and his little nephew, George.

Ash looked like a kid in a sweetshop. I lost him about ten times, only to find him drooling over an old Ferrari as if it was a leggy blonde. He's such a boy. It was boiling hot that day, and I'd rather have been looking at shoes but, frankly, I couldn't have been happier. I was just like everyone else. I was delighted to be doing normal things.

It was funny walking into the chemo ward on 22 August for what I hoped would be the final time. My friend Alison was accompanying me, and we'd brought cake, which we distributed to the nurses and other patients on the ward.

I couldn't quite believe that we had at last reached this point. Session six of my chemo marked the very welcome end of the worst and most difficult chapter of my life. Everything had seemed so impossible when I went for my first session – how could I ever get through being diagnosed with cancer? How could I deal with all those chemo sessions? But I had. I'd bloody done it!

It seemed like an eternity since I'd faced the devastating news that I had breast cancer. But, in reality, it had been just four months earlier, in April, when Gigi was just ten weeks old.

As the nurses plugged me in for the final time, I felt triumphant. It's amazing how you can cope when you have to. It had often felt like my world was falling apart, and the chemo was nothing short of hideous, but I'd found my own coping mechanism. What other choice did I have?

I had my war wounds – a lumpectomy scar, no hair, a face bloated by the steroids for the chemo, I'd put on weight (and I knew it could take up to a year to get rid of the toxins) – but I felt very optimistic that I could get back to normal fast.

When my final session was over, I hugged the nurses goodbye.

'No offence, but I really hope I NEVER see you again,' I joked.

Then I was off, stepping outside into the unseasonably crisp air of that cold and rainy August 2008.

Autumn was just around the corner, and I felt excited. There was a feeling of change in the air. The leaves on the trees would soon turn brown, red and gold, and the kids would be heading back to school.

But, best of all, my chemo was over. Things were looking up . . .

9. Ash's Chapter

When I met Rebekah, I knew that life would never be dull, but even I had no idea that our introduction to parenthood would be so dramatic. Ten weeks after watching my lovely fiancée push our daughter into the world, when most couples have just about got the new arrival into some kind of routine, I was faced with the fact that Rebekah had cancer and could die.

The birth itself was magical; without doubt, the happiest day of my life. There was Beck, me, and my sister in the birthing room, and then our beautiful girl, Gisele Amber Pitman, arrived. Previously, the plan had been for me to wait outside – Beck was worried that seeing the birth would be too much for me, that it might put me off her! She spent so much of the pregnancy worrying about everything that could go wrong (it drove me slightly mad!), and I know that included how I would cope with it all.

I have to admit that I wasn't too upset when she told me that her mum would be her birthing partner – I hadn't been to any antenatal classes, but I had plenty of mates who had relayed their horror stories, and none of it sounded good! I certainly wasn't surprised that Beck took charge of the pregnancy and birthing plans – that's the way she has always been. She thrives on giving me the impression she is in control at all times; it's part of our dynamic: Beck out there on the front line and me in the background passing the ammunition, giving her the confidence talks when she falters, bolstering her when she needs it – although cancer changed that, and our roles reversed for a time. I have come to realize that you can't be diagnosed with cancer one day and be the same person afterwards. I'm not the same as I was, so God knows how you cope when it's you who is facing your own mortality. Cancer diagnosis was the first time in sixteen years that the mask came off and I saw Beck at a loss.

When I look back to Gigi's birth, it's proof things happen for a reason. Cancer or not, having been there by Rebekah's side, I wouldn't have it any other way, but that feeling was more intense once she had been diagnosed – it was all the more important for me to have seen my little girl being born. Someone had to be able to pass on the moment if Rebekah wasn't going to be around.

The whole birth went like clockwork. The sun was shining and, suddenly, our daughter was there, and staring at everything around her. Nothing can quite prepare you for seeing your baby take in the world for the very first time, and we were both bowled over. Showing my newborn little girl to my mum and dad was a proud moment I will treasure for ever.

From the moment I saw Rebekah with Gigi, I knew she was born to be a mum. I know she claims to have been nervous, and she was overwhelmed for a while, but she took to motherhood like a duck to water. As my mum said as soon as she arrived at the hospital and saw them together, 'She's a natural, that one.'

I loved having our own little family – my relationship with Beck felt deeper and more complete. I was the proudest man around. The love you have for your child is like no other, you would do anything for them and, during the birth, my admiration for Rebekah soared. But, when I look back at those fantastic first weeks, all I can think is 'Beck has cancer.' The whole time we were marvelling at what we had created, cancer was igniting, travelling and threatening to snatch it all away. It had been there all along, lurking in the background and waiting until it could rear its ugly head and screw up our lives.

The agonizing thing is that, deep down, as soon as Rebekah found that lump just before Christmas, I knew something was wrong and, when I think back, I feel incredibly guilty. As soon as she made me run my hand over the swelling, I knew it wasn't good news. I knew what a lump in the breast could mean.

I told her it would be fine, but that she should go straight to the doctor. That night, we both went to bed feeling scared. I remember lying there and giving myself a good talking to: 'Don't be an idiot, Ash. Who the hell gets cancer when they are pregnant?'

When she came back on Christmas Eve, grinning and reiterating that her GP had said it was a blocked milk duct, I still had an uneasy feeling. After initially sharing her joy at the 'all clear', the fear settled back in. But I'm not a doctor, and Rebekah was heavily pregnant and hormonal. She'd made such an effort to be healthy for our baby – I know how hard she worked at giving Gigi the best start in life – and the thought of people prodding, poking and invading that cocoon she'd created for Gigi terrified her. Who was I to tell her she was wrong? In reality, I needed to believe it was fine as much as she did. The last thing I wanted to do was upset her, so I reminded myself that she'd had a professional all clear and tried to forget about it.

Only I couldn't.

I think I really began to feel alarmed after Gigi was born in February and the lump was still there. I kept thinking, If that was a blocked milk duct, it would be bigger or smaller by now. Surely Gigi wouldn't be feeding so well? There's got to be something more to this, but first-time parenthood is all-consuming and, although Beck did most of the work, we were both shell-shocked and exhausted.

Looking back, I get so cross that I didn't insist she go back to the doctor. I don't know why I didn't. It didn't help that Beck is normally so in control, so, when she lost her confidence after the baby was born, my main concern was that she didn't slip into postnatal depression. She was weepy, and everything seemed like the biggest challenge. She struggled to leave the house, and alarm bells were ringing in my head. You hear terrible stories of women being taken over by depression after giving birth, how it can wreck everything and change a woman for ever. It's ironic that we already had devastation coming our way, but in a different form.

But then Rebekah went to see the locum doctor, who gave her another all clear, plus, she had a referral appointment booked. She had seen two GPs who weren't even slightly concerned, so why did I have this sense of impending doom? I was worried that being a father had turned me into a perpetual worrier, so I did my best to rein it in.

The turning point came when we went to Spain in March. Rebekah's hospital referral was three weeks away. And then *bang!* My close mate, Richard, called my mobile to say that his wife, Madeleine, had breast cancer. It was a total blow.

Richard was heart-broken. He was so shocked that this was happening to them. Madeleine was healthy and young – but then, so was Rebekah. I couldn't believe what I was hearing, I was gutted for them both. They were a golden couple who had everything going for them, good people who didn't deserve this. It was awful to hear my friend contemplating the worst. As I went into overdrive, doling out clichéd reassurances to Richard and promising him and Madeleine all the support I could offer, I couldn't stop thinking about Rebekah. Talking about someone we knew having cancer made our own situation all too real.

A light went on: I know Rebekah has cancer, I thought. After we had talked through what was next for Madeleine and how the doctors were going to treat it, I took a deep breath and confided my fears to Richard:

'Listen, mate, I'm really concerned about Rebekah,' I said. 'She's got a lump, too. She's had it since Christmas.'

Richard seemed unconvinced. 'Come on, she'll be fine,' he said. 'What are the chances of it happening to both of them at their age?'

We went on reassuring each other it would all be OK, and Richard decided he wouldn't tell Madeleine about Rebekah – more stress and upset was the last thing she needed. We signed off with me promising him a pint when we were back, and I hung up. I took a deep breath and told Rebekah about Madeleine. She was inconsolable. To be honest, it was the reaction I'd wanted: to shock her into understanding how serious this was. And it worked.

'The moment that plane touches down, you're going to the doctor's. That's it,' I told her, frowning. I'd had enough of her being passed from pillar to post. It was time to have some tests and find out for sure what was going on.

So, when we landed at Gatwick two days later, the first thing I said as we unstrapped our seatbelts was, 'Remember, you're going to the doctor's.'

'Yes,' she sighed. 'I will. Promise.'

I was really militant with her all week, but I could tell she was delaying. The final straw was after I had been to the pub with Richard. I came home, realized Rebekah still hadn't made an appointment, and I lost it with her. I was terrified we were facing the same fate as Richard and Madeleine. I told her she had to get it seen to and that I wouldn't speak to her until she had. It had the desired effect but, when she did finally get an appointment with her GP, I phoned her up beforehand, and we had another row.

'Make sure you demand that referral. You shouldn't have to wait another day, Rebekah,' I insisted. 'Just tell them we'll pay for it.'

'Why are you freaking out?' she shouted defensively. 'For Christ's sake, I can deal with it. Just because Madeleine has breast cancer, it doesn't mean I have.' I know she was as scared as me; we've spoken about how we were feeling since and confided that we both feared it was bad news. Becks didn't want to burst our bubble by knowing for definite and having to deal with it. She was terrified.

From the moment she went to the surgery, everything turned crazy. Things went from her GP being worried to her appointment with Mr Williams, who was convinced the lump was suspicious. I will never forget taking that phone call from Rebekah, hearing those words: 'They think it's cancer. Mr Williams said he'll be very surprised if it's not malignant.' I just wanted to shout, 'Don't say that. What the hell do you mean?'

I felt as if I'd been hit in the gut with a baseball bat. I couldn't believe this was really happening to us. Nothing will ever be the same again, I thought. But I immediately went into a role of being positive. We'd had our normality snatched away. This was it – my partner could die, but she needed me to step up and be strong.

'Lots of people get cancer and get over it,' I told her. 'Come home, Beck, and we'll talk it through, and it will be OK.' But she was inconsolable. I grabbed my keys ready to fetch her and Gigi, but she was insistent she could drive herself. And so began the walking on eggshells – of course I wanted to pick her up, but she didn't want me to, and I had to respect that. I had no choice but to follow her lead – it was Rebekah who had the cancer, after all.

When I put the phone down, I was devastated. You never imagine you'll be in that position – there's no training for your life partner getting cancer at thirty-five.

I called my mum and dad in Spain. By now, my guard was down, and nothing they could say could make things any better. They were gutted too and arranged to come home on the next plane.

Then I rang Amber, and she assumed that supportive role, telling me calmly about her mates who had had it, and their mums who had been through it. 'It'll all be fine,' she said. 'Beck is a fighter, Ash.'

I still think hearing for the first time that Rebekah probably had cancer has remained one of the worst moments. It's a total fear of the unknown. But, as we got further into the cancer system, things got worse.

The day Rebekah had the ultrasound, I waited by the phone with the baby while she attended the appointment with Charlotte. Even then she was more concerned about interrupting Gigi's routine – another example of what a wonderful mother she is: our daughter has always come first.

I waited for two hours. It was the longest wait of my life, an eternity.

Of course, by then, we already knew things didn't look good. Mr Williams had been matter-of-fact about his thoughts – he was pretty sure it was cancer.

I kept telling myself that there was a small chance she didn't have it. Right up to the official diagnosis, I always had hope, praying for those small odds to come our way. But then Rebekah phoned and told me they really were sure: 'It's breast cancer. That's it.' She was crying so much I could hardly understand what she was saying.

When I called Richard, he just couldn't believe it, that what had happened to Madeleine was now happening to Rebekah. Now we both had partners with breast cancer. What a crap bond to share.

Everyone was speechless. It sounds trite, but this shit completely changes the way you look at life. You don't look ahead in decades, but hours, days and weeks. I'd never examined my own mortality or thought about Rebekah's but, now, I found myself thinking, Jesus, Rebekah might only have five years, or The baby is so tiny – will Rebekah be dead by the time she's walking? Will I be bringing up our daughter alone?

I couldn't even begin to imagine how I'd do it, how I'd ever cope. Would Rebekah even be given the chance to leave a mark on our little girl? Would she have time to impart some influence on her daughter, or would Gigi grow up not remembering her, with only memory boxes to open when she wanted to spend time with her mummy? Of course, the biggest hope then and now is that we'll look back in ten years' time and say, 'Thank God we got through that.'

I felt numb. This was the biggest thing we had ever faced, and there was nothing I could do to fix it. I hated feeling so helpless when my family was at stake.

Despite the dark thoughts, however, I can remember thinking when she came back with Charlotte that day that I had to be upbeat. Something just happened in my head, and I wanted to protect her. My 'front' went on. I couldn't let her see my fear, it wouldn't help anything.

Rebekah was crushed. I gave her a big hug and told her, 'We will fight this. Together.'

I switched straight into pragmatic mode, asking Charlotte exactly what had been said, if there were any notes for me to look at, what the next step was, when Rebekah was seeing the doctor again.

Rebekah sat there looking blank. She looked as numb as I felt. She was petrified, so I tried to give the impression I wasn't thinking the worst, even though all sorts of awful scenarios were flying through my mind. We couldn't both fold. Someone had to be strong.

From the very moment of Rebekah's diagnosis, the main aim was to have her treated, draw a line under it and get on with our lives as quickly as possible. But I had no idea how long that torturous diagnosis period would go on for. From the first doctor's appointment, to waiting to see what surgery and treatment she would need, to the operation itself, and then the hideous wait to see if the cancer had spread. The whole period took four months. It felt like a prison sentence.

We took some really bad knocks early on. When they did the biopsy and the cancer-specialist nurse told us that Rebekah had grade-three cancer, all I wanted to know was, Is she going to live? I wasn't even sure if there was a grade four. We knew Madeleine had grade two, and I remembered someone telling me, 'As long as she hasn't got the worst grade, she'll be cured.'

But Rebekah did have the worst grade – it didn't get any more depressing than grade-three – and I came away from that appointment feeling we were fighting an impossible fight. I felt defeated before we'd even begun.

Rebekah looked to me for constant reassurance, and I always tried to give it to her. I encouraged her to keep off the internet, not to look up facts, figures and statistics that would make her feel any more down. I begged her to concentrate on what she could do, what she could change. The irony was that, while I was encouraging her to be totally positive, I was finding out all I could.

Those few days after her diagnosis were my angriest time. I was holding it together at home but, inside, I was raging. I felt useless. I've always been the one to make it all OK, my role is to protect Rebekah, to offer the solutions, and here I was, unable to do anything but hope for the best. Rebekah coped by throwing herself into looking after Gigi. She wouldn't let me do anything to help, which was frustrating, as that was something I could have done to lighten the load. One day, I broke down. I couldn't help myself, but I realized by the look on Rebekah's face that it didn't change things, and it didn't help her.

I remember driving to work another day and losing control. It all came pouring out. 'What the f**k has Rebekah done to deserve this?' I kept asking myself. I can remember roaring at the top of my voice in a traffic jam, and banging the steering wheel and weeping. The driver in the car to my right looked bemused by my outburst, but those trips to work became something of a routine, time to deal with how I was feeling. I was as angry, scared and desperate as Rebekah was.

In the build-up to her operation, I got a crash course in the stark reality of cancer and the fact that there are no quick fixes or answers. At every turn, I'd be desperate to ask, 'Is she going to survive this? What are her chances?' The thing was, though, that there is no definitive answer.

You assume you won't cope. Then, time passes and you start ticking things off the list and thinking, Maybe we *could* get out of this! – but then something else happens to set you back. Taking Rebekah in for the surgery nearly killed me, especially watching her sign the papers granting the surgeon permission to remove anything else if the cancer had spread. Kissing her goodbye was so hard, she was petrified as she was taken to theatre, and it did flash through my mind that it could be the last time I would see her.

I was determined not to allow Rebekah to think that cancer was going to kill her. It was always, You're going to beat this cancer, have this operation, take this pill, pump these drugs into your veins and it will be fine. It was all about being positive.

The fact that Rebekah chose to believe everything I said has been a blessing and a curse throughout this period. Telling her what she needs to hear has been draining at times. It's made me feel uneasy and superstitious, as if I am somehow tempting fate.

One of the most difficult times was when I knew the cancer had probably spread to the lymph nodes and decided to keep it from Rebekah to protect her.

After she had the lumpectomy, I asked to see Mr Williams while she was still coming round from the anaesthetic. He was so hectic that I ended up catching him in the corridor. I could tell by looking at him he wasn't pleased and I begged him to tell me what had happened during the op, what he thought, off the record. I needed to know the worst. In the end I had to force it out of him.

'I've taken the lump out, and I've done an axillary clearance of Rebekah's lymph nodes,' he explained.

'How do you think it went?' I asked. 'Has it spread?'

'I can only tell you what I think,' he replied. 'I've taken all the lymphs out and several, in my opinion, were tumorous.'

My heart sank. 'What, cancerous?' I asked.

'I would be surprised if they weren't,' he confirmed.

I was gutted. It was exactly what we didn't want to hear. We wanted a perfect little lump that could be cut away leaving no trace. I'd heard the stories about lymph nodes helping cancer spread around the body. I knew it could be fatal.

I felt broken, sitting in reception wondering what I should do, thinking, Where else is it? Where's it going next?

I rang Mum and Dad. I had to tell someone. They were floored, too, and found it difficult to tell me everything would be OK. We all knew it sounded like the end. After a while, I managed to get hold of Amber and, once again, she was strong for me.

'It's a blow, but it's not the end of the world, Ash,' she said, being rational. 'Just wait and see what the results are before you get yourself into a state.' Her stoic attitude reminded me I needed to get it together before Rebekah came round.

I was outside in the waiting room for an hour trying to pull myself together, weighing up my options. The news had devastated me – God knows what it would do to Beck after having such a massive operation. I couldn't tell her. It was dreadful to imagine concealing something so huge from her, but what option did I have? This was life and death, and I had no idea how to handle it. In the end, I just went with my gut feeling and told her it was all fine.

Some people might think it's strange, keeping such important news to myself, but I know Beck. She had come this far by focusing on what she could do to beat the cancer, by building up a wall of positivity and telling herself she was in control. Telling her it had spread would be acknowledging that the disease had a life of its own and that no amount of hard work and treatment could change things. She would have been crushed. She had to believe that the operation was the beginning of the fight rather than the end of her hope.

She needs to get strong again, I decided. We'll wait for a definitive answer and, in the meantime, I'll say nothing.

I went back into Beck's room. She had come round after the operation. 'How are you feeling?' I asked.

'OK,' she said, looking down at her chest anxiously to see if they'd had to do more surgery than they'd planned.

Three or four hours went past before she finally said, 'Did you see the doctor?'

She looked worried. She was frightened to ask, and it confirmed to me that I was doing the right thing not telling her. So I simply said, 'Mr Williams thinks it all went well.'

It was a bare-faced lie, but I could see that she was relieved.

It was a lonely time for me – knowing what was coming and continuing to pretend all was well and that we'd had the best possible news. *She* was supposed to be the one who was good at acting! But I now know she wasn't convinced, she was clutching at straws and taking me at my word.

Later, I felt haunted and asked Maggie, the nurse at the Spire, if I could have a word with her when Rebekah was sleeping.

'Have you spoken to Mr Williams?' I asked.

'Yes. I know as much as there is to know,' she replied.

'I'm almost frightened to ask you,' I started to say, my throat tightening with the threat of tears. All at once, I was too choked to speak.

She was a lovely lady. She leaned across and held my hand. 'Just ask, and I'll go through it with you,' she said.

'What does this mean, about it being in the lymph

nodes?' I eventually managed to splutter.

'I don't know for sure,' she replied.

'But hypothetically?' I pleaded.

'It's the highway to the body,' she answered.

I then asked what the procedure would be. Maggie explained that they would give Rebekah a scan and do 'staging' to see how far the cancer had gone into her body.

This was much more serious than I had thought it would be.

Maggie interrupted my melancholy musings. 'I'm just telling you the worst-case scenario,' she said softly. 'She might not need scans or staging.'

I tried to smile, thanking her for her time, but I felt so low. My world was crumbling around me.

It transpired that she'd need all that, and more. But I kept my chats with both Mr Williams and Maggie quiet. What Rebekah didn't know couldn't hurt her.

I did phone Rebekah's mum to tell her the news about the lymph nodes. Rebekah was her daughter, after all, and she had a right to know. I imagined being in the same position with Gigi, and someone making that decision on her behalf. It didn't bear thinking about. 'I'm not telling her yet,' I warned Rebekah's mum. 'And I don't want any talk about her dying. We need to be as positive as possible and assume it'll be OK.'

Maybe it was out of order to speak to her mum like that, but I wanted to make sure we were all in agreement about what was best. I wanted us to build Rebekah's confidence. I couldn't take the suffering away from her, but I felt that this was the only constructive way I could help her through it, by getting her strong for the next stage.

For all the positivity I was encouraging in her and the people around her, however, inside, my own thoughts were shockingly morbid. On that first post-op night at my mum's house, I started thinking how I could make it work if Rebekah was taken from me. How would I bring up our daughter? Would I have a nanny? Was that what Rebekah would want? Would I move in with my parents? How would I ever smile again without my beautiful, witty Beck? I hated thinking like this, but I couldn't help it, those dark thoughts chipped away at me late at night – and still do, to tell the honest truth.

As well as all the practical stuff, I found myself contemplating deeper issues: Would I ever meet someone else, would I love her like Rebekah, or would I mess up any potential relationship because I'd always put Gigi first? If I was straight with myself, I knew I probably would.

The silly thing is, Rebekah and I had discussed this stuff before but, ironically, it had always been the reverse scenario. Because I was the older one and had the stressful job working for the family business and could rarely take time off, I'd always said, 'If something happens to me, make sure you get someone who loves you and cares for you. Go for someone who can look after you.'

'I'm going to make a play for Simon Cowell,' she'd joke. All our chats were about something happening to me, so it was weird to sit and think about what I'd do if Rebekah died. What I would do if that light went out. What I did know is that our daughter would always come first, she would be Rebekah's legacy, even if she would be slightly indulged with lots of pink ponies! I would cope, I'd do it for Beck. We'd already agreed on how we would bring her up, on the things that were important.

I didn't really have a lot of time to wallow in thoughts like this, though, as, in the days after the surgery, we got a taste of just how life-changing cancer was, especially when Rebekah's dressing leaked.

Rebekah was stressed and angry that our lives had been interrupted and was clinging on to the hope that her lymphs would be clear. I kept the news from her until the day we went back to see Mr Williams, but I knew I had to prepare her for the news somehow.

'There is a possibility it might have gone into your lymphs,' I said, broaching the subject with her in the car on the way there.

But Rebekah was having none of it. 'No, I'm sure it hasn't,' she said. Clearly, all that positive thinking was working.

'If it has, it's not a big deal,' I continued. 'There are plenty of people who have survived. It's just another hurdle.'

I don't think it really sank in for her until Mr Williams told her that nineteen of her thirty-three glands were affected. She was devastated. The colour drained from her face. She could tell from my reaction that I must have known, but I had always been confident she'd understand I kept it from her to protect her. It's not exactly news you'd relish keeping to yourself for any other reason.

We already knew it was a particularly aggressive cancer, but Mr Williams took the time to explain to us again.

'What does it mean for us now?' I asked.

'It means we have to give Rebekah more protection,' he said. 'Maybe the body has done a good job of acting as a filtering system or, possibly, it has already spread. We need to find out with the scans.'

Then it got worse. If I think back to that time, all I remember is Beck looking haunted. It was heart-breaking to see. She got through it a bit at a time. I tried to make her feel as upbeat as I could, even if that meant constantly putting a positive spin on bad news. We were fighting for survival, and I'd deal with the consequences later.

We had dozens of conversations when I'd come home from work and she would be crying, or she would wake up in the middle of the night convinced she was dying. The night before her scan was particularly awful, and one of the few times my mask slipped, as I held her and told her how much I loved her. We both cried for all that was at stake.

I'd always listen to her fears and then reassure her she would be fine. She would ask me how I could remain so positive, so sure everything would be fine, and I would say the same thing: 'I'm telling you, you'll be fine. I know it.'

At the time, I felt like a fraud. But, if Rebekah had been able to read my mind, it would have broken her. I was crippled by the fear that I could lose her, but she didn't need to know that. Being frightened of what was happening with her own body was enough for her to cope with.

Throughout all this, Richard was brilliant – he was the only person who knew how it felt to watch your partner fighting to live. He knew how much was at stake with every appointment and scan. We had regular get-togethers. Sometimes we didn't mention cancer at all but talked around it. Whatever we discussed, those times were a lifeline for me. Other mates rallied round, too. I went for a coffee with one friend a couple of days before Rebekah's first bone scan, and we were talking about Rebekah's prognosis.

'I'm terrified that the cancer is everywhere. It could be in any part of her body,' I confided to him, and then I started to cry. I was exhausted from hiding my fears. When I let it all out, I saw him well up. Once we'd both finished, he patted me on the back and said, 'Jesus, I feel really done in!'

'Yeah, I feel like that all the time,' I replied. 'And there's no escape from it.'

The morning Rebekah had the first scan, I went with her. It was further confirmation that we were part of something huge, and there was no running away. We were in a place with really sick people. That waiting room was rammed with people from all walks of life. Some had no hair, some had tubes everywhere, some were young, some old, some just babies. All I could think about was our little Gigi, and the tears started to come. There was a whole spectrum of humanity here, and that included Beck.

Rebekah had to drink a massive jug of liquid contrast, and then she had the scan. That night, waiting for the results, was horrendous. While Rebekah had a bath, I picked up Gigi from her cot (even though she was asleep!) and held her close. What would we do if it was more bad news? I didn't sleep at all that night, preparing myself for the worst, that the cancer had spread to the liver and beyond.

The next morning I had to go to work, so Rebekah went back to the hospital with Charlotte to have her next bone scan. She was also eagerly awaiting a call that would deliver the restults of her first scan.

I was at the garage when she phoned to say that it had come back clear. I can still remember exactly where I was in the car yard when I answered my mobile. I leapt around like I'd won the lottery. It was a feeling of pure elation.

One of the guys who works with us looked up and shouted, 'What is it?'

'Her scan is clear,' I yelled. Everyone there knew what had been going on and, soon, they were all whooping with glee too. We were thrilled.

Thank God both scans came back clear. It was an unbelievable relief and, for me, it marked a clear turning point. I allowed myself to feel hope for the first time.

But I also thought about all those people we'd seen sitting in the oncology waiting room. The law of averages meant that, for all those waiting their turn for tests and consultations, there would be as many receiving bad news as good.

We clung on to the good and celebrated Rebekah's news before preparing ourselves for the next challenge – her course of chemotherapy. This was when my resolve was seriously tested. It was a bleak, bleak time and, during it, we both felt like giving up more than once. I watched her be taken to the brink by the treatment, and it was hard to keep remembering that they had to do that before they could bring her back. I read that hideous leaflet detailing the possible side effects of something that was being administered to cure her and felt I was in a horror film. At times, it was as if they were killing her, as they dripped more and more poison into her system.

When Rebekah started her chemo and her hair began to fall out, I felt incredibly sad for her. Her glossy barnet was so much a part of who she was, and I had always loved it.

Losing her hair was the thing that preoccupied her – it acted as a distraction from all the other side effects. I know she felt I didn't have a clue what she was going through, especially with something as huge to her as her hair loss. Perhaps I didn't always understand, but the point I always tried to make was that losing her locks was a good thing. It was the sign we needed to know that the treatment was working, attacking and killing all the fast-multiplying cells. My philosophy was, the quicker your hair goes, the quicker the drugs are working, so, in a strange way, the sicker she was, the happier I felt.

In the end, she decided to shave all her hair off, and that was so empowering for her. Seeing Beck bald for the first time took my breath away; she'd never looked more beautiful.

But before all that, going with Rebekah for her first chemo session was frightening. The nurses were all really supportive from the start, and Rebekah became really friendly with them. They do the most amazing job. That first session, she was so nervous and, as they explained about the drug – what it was doing and how she could expect to feel – I swear she looked like she was going to do a runner! But, once the treatment had begun and the initial session was out of the way, she was really brave. That first one really disturbed me. I looked over at her half way through it and saw that she'd changed colour. Her skin looked really flushed, with a big red line. It was as though your eyes were following the chemo as it coursed around her veins. Just like those we had seen in the bone scan waiting room, lots of the people having treatment alongside Beck looked tired, ill and had lost their hair. In comparison, Rebekah was really glamorous, with her long hair and make-up. But, as the weeks went on, she began to look like everyone else – no hair, grey and yellow in equal measure, and really unwell – as though she was slowly being poisoned.

Her eyes were jaundiced, her teeth looked grey, as if they were about to fall out, and she had days when she couldn't lift her head from the pillow. At times like that, my mum was a saint and stepped in to look after the baby, while Rebekah tried to sleep as much as she could.

I think that, other than at the time of the diagnosis, this was when I felt most useless. Rebekah's moods would change in the snap of a finger. I couldn't do anything right. Everything annoyed her, and I had to learn tolerance fast. Throughout our relationship we'd always had fights – we both loved to clear the air with a good ruck. But, this time, as she sniped and raged at me, I just had to take it – she was being violently sick, she looked so frail and ill, there was no way I could give as good as I got. Nothing was normal, least of all our relationship. She insisted on business as usual when it came to Gigi, and then got upset that she was doing it all on her own. I didn't know which Beck would greet me when I came home from work and my job became a bit of an escape from it all.

But whatever Rebekah's mood, I felt so protective of her. There were times at night when I'd wake up and stare at her. She looked so fragile and sick it felt as if she was disintegrating before my eyes. I wondered what we would do if the cancer came back – could her body cope with a second round of chemo? Could we? She got really depressed. I remember coming home one day and catching her watching an episode of *Casualty* on UK Gold. It must have been awful seeing herself in her glamorous prime, looking amazing and doing what she loved when, now, she felt so crap, had no hair and was fighting to survive. I had to look away. But, to me, she has always been beautiful, and I hope I have told her that throughout the cancer as much as she has needed to hear it.

Her girlfriends have been a godsend. They've all rallied and helped with Gigi, and I've seen first hand how much that support has helped Beck and, in turn, me. It goes without saying that my mum has been amazing – we owe her and my dad so much as well as Rebekah's parents and their partners. And our neighbour, Victoria, was fabulous. It was she who did the shopping, washing and ironing when Beck couldn't even get dressed. But what I am most grateful for is the way that Victoria helped Rebekah through the depression that hit during the treatment. Bit by bit, she opened up the world again for Beck. She went from not being able to leave her bed to wandering down the road for a coffee. A few weeks later, they were heading into town for some lunch and a spot of shopping, and Rebekah didn't even realize she'd overcome such a huge hurdle. That is testament to Victoria's love, care and laidback attitude.

There were also important discussions to be had, especially when it came to the prospect of having more children. We had been told in no uncertain terms that chemotherapy can hinder fertility, and it forced our hand when it came to discussing the future. For me, it was never a big issue to have more children. We have the most incredible daughter, she's the light of our lives. In some ways, we are no different from any other couple. Who says, just because you have had one child, you'll be able to have another? There are all sorts of things that can conspire against you, and we are luckier than some, who can't have any children, who invest all that hope and money in IVF only to be disappointed. We are experiencing the joy of parenthood with our beloved Gigi, and I thank God for her every day. Having researched further, I can't help but worry that if you have developed cancer once while pregnant, there could be a very real chance of it happening again. Your hormones are flying, and the body is in shock as it copes with giving something else life – I don't ever want to put Beck in that danger.

I had followed Rebekah's lead (like most men, I reckon!) when it came to deciding the time was right to have Gigi – partly as I knew how much it meant to her. But I wanted it too: I wanted a family, and now we have one. I don't need to go through it again. We've tested our luck once, and I can't begin to imagine how we would have coped with the cancer if we hadn't already had Gigi. I don't know that Rebekah could have.

I prefer to count my blessings and enjoy what we have. I don't even want to contemplate taking a risk with Rebekah once she's in remission but, if she really wants another baby of her own, then she's had all the implants to help protect her ovaries, and we will discuss it. We might be a partnership, but it's her body and I have to respect that. We always talked about having a gaggle of kids, a big and noisy family, everyone with their own personalities but, if that's meant to be, then we will try to adopt. It was never the plan that Gigi would be an only child; we didn't want that. But this is the hand we have been dealt.

Adoption is a real possibility, especially as my mum was in a children's home. I think we have a lot to give, and Rebekah is an outstanding mother. Any child would be lucky to have her. For now, though, my focus is entirely on getting her well and preserving what we have. Extending our family is the least of my worries.

The scary times continued with regularity. One of the most frightening episodes was when Rebekah reacted to the anti-sickness drug and her jaw locked. I thought she was dying.

She was gurning and had lost any control of her jaw, which meant her tongue was hanging out of her mouth.

We called the chemo helpline, but they didn't know what was wrong and advised us to call an ambulance.

We were taken to A&E, and it was absolute chaos – car crashes, drunk people, fight victims: a typical Saturday night.

Rebekah was lying there on a bed looking dazed and bewildered as they decided that she'd had an allergic reaction to the anti-sickness drugs. The nurses knew what medication they needed to administer, but they had trouble trying to get hold of the right drug. It turned out the on-call pharmacist lived twenty to thirty miles away, and they kept calling him for advice. Rather than making the long trek to the hospital, he kept sending them on a wild-goose chase round the hospital, looking for this bloody medication. They'd call him and say, 'No it's not on ward 6. Where else should we try?' And he'd reply, 'Try the theatre ward.'

Well, after two hours, I lost the plot. Rebekah looked so vulnerable and unwell, like she was fitting, and I nearly cried at such a loss of dignity for her, to be lying in hospital with cancer, being mucked around for a drug she should have been given the minute she arrived. I demanded to see the consultant in charge, and I didn't mince my words. 'Never mind the fact that my fiancée could DIE here, on a basic management level, you're doing something wrong,' I told her. 'You're paying someone to be on duty, so do me a favour and get that person in.'

To her credit, she said, 'No, you're completely right,' and

then instructed the nurses to get back on the phone and demand that the pharmacist come in.

Within an hour, he'd arrived and had administered the drug she needed. She was fixed within half an hour after that. I felt so angry – how pointless was it to just have her sitting in casualty in that state because they couldn't give her a drug that was locked in a room downstairs? It beggared belief.

Anger was a bit of a theme for me at this point, and never more than when Beck insisted on taking part in the Race for Life. She was so sick, her temperature was sky-high and, yet, no matter how much I begged her to pull out, Beck insisted on fulfilling her commitments. When we had to go to A&E for the second time in a week, I was angry with her for being so stubborn. I was barely speaking to her. But, the truth of the matter is, once I knew she was OK, I thought, That's my girl, a fighter. Her courage amazed me, even if I did get cross when she wouldn't do as she was told!

The final chemo sessions were hard for me, too, to know that she had taken all the drugs she could and that now it was up to fate – well, that made me feel more helpless than ever.

I like to think that the darkest times have passed; Rebekah has finished her chemotherapy and completed a course of radiotherapy too. The latter was less invasive than the chemo but just as draining, and it meant we had some more tough times as she battled with extreme tiredness.

But now all the invasive treatment is over, she's getting on with her life, taking it a day at a time – looking after the baby, going out for walks and seeing her friends. She and Gigi always look immaculate, Gigi in one of her hundreds of outfits and Beck with her lipgloss and high heels on. Most of all, she is positive and upbeat.

To say that I am in awe of her is an understatement. She's been amazing throughout this ordeal and has done 99 per cent of it on her own.

Every day, I pray she's going to be fine, that we will enjoy our grandchildren together and do all the things we planned. But my cautious nature also tells me not to assume anything – who'd have thought she would get cancer in the first place? There's still a tiny part of me that thinks about the 'what if', what I will do if it's just me and Gigi, but I try not to think about it, not to manufacture those conversations where you casually mention that you would prefer to be buried rather than cremated and wait for the reply, to log away in your mind for the day it might be needed.

What I find hard is watching her add to the memory boxes she created for Gigi. She continues to collect all sorts of stuff, anything that tells a story about who she is, in case that is all our daughter has, and that kills me. When I think back to how I laughed at Beck when she started collecting odds and ends for the boxes while she was pregnant, the irony isn't lost on me. Who'd have thought we would ever need them? But we have to face the fact that we might, after all, and I know that's as close as either of us can come to admitting she might die.

The whole battle has changed me. I have become really emotional, for a start. If I begin to describe what Beck has been through, I get really choked up. But, most of all, I have vowed to make the most of what I have got. I had Rebekah for all those years when I wasn't sure about making a commitment, wasn't sure what I wanted and, when I had finally taken the plunge and we were living a dream existence, cancer struck and I nearly lost everything.

I am so proud of Beck – her guts, her strength and courage – and if ever there is any testament to her fighting spirit, it's Gigi. She is a complete joy. I worried constantly about how the cancer would affect her, if all the stress and Beck being ill would leave its mark, but she has had so much love from everyone, she is unscathed. Something positive has come out of something so hideous, and that is all to Rebekah's credit. Our daughter is always laughing and taking pleasure in the smallest things. She's such a product of Rebekah.

It's definitely made me realize that everything in life is finite. Rebekah might have one year left, or sixty. She could be in remission until she is ninety, or the cancer could come back next year. I've never really thought like that before, I was too busy chipping along trying to pay off the mortgage and keep on top of the credit cards. Beck being ill has made me stop and smell the roses. We are bombarded with tales of cancer, new wonder drugs and pioneering surgery and, although it might lodge somewhere in the back of your brain, you never imagine cancer will affect you or the person you adore.

But it has, and I know first hand how fragile life is. I feel so lucky to have been given a second chance with such a phenomenal woman. I'll be proud to call her my wife.

10. A Second Chance

I was at home in the shower when I felt another lump in my breast.

The scar from my lumpectomy was feeling quite painful, so I ran my finger over it. It instantly made me recoil. There, beneath the skin, was a weird little lump, kind of grizzly and the size of a five-pence piece. It was right next to the scar where the cancerous tumour had been removed four months earlier. Finding it there made me feel physically sick. I don't want another lump, I thought. I don't have the energy.

Once your chemo was over, I noticed that people tended to assume that that was it: job done.

'Oh, you're at the end,' one friend would say. 'Your hair is growing back!'

'Is that it then?' someone else would comment. 'Are you in remission?'

Whenever conversations like this occurred, all I really wanted to do was bat the few eyelashes that had grown back in disbelief and rant, 'Actually, this nightmare is far from over. I thought finishing chemo would make me feel serene, but I feel really angry inside. Just because I look a little less sick doesn't mean I'm cured. Just because I've sprouted a couple of millimetres of hair doesn't mean the cancer's gone. In fact, I won't know if I've beaten cancer for a long time yet and, right now, there are a million additional things to worry about. I still need ECGs, bloodtests. I look for moles, if there's a pain in my chest I worry. If I've got the runs, I wonder if it will make my tablets less effective . . . Cancer still consumes my every waking hour.'

But outbursts like this, to well-meaning people kindly enquiring after your health, are not the done thing, are they? So, instead, I found myself smiling politely and replying, 'Actually, not quite. I've still got another year until I'm really through it, unfortunately.'

Finding another lump scared the shit out of me.

'Ash,' I shouted. 'Come and see this.'

He rushed into the bathroom, a look of concern on his face.

'Give me your hand,' I instructed, then I took his finger and showed him where the lump was.

Like me, he immediately recoiled. 'I can't touch it,' he said. But then he did put his hand back and ran his finger over it. 'It's probably nothing,' he soothed, 'but you need to call Rema now to see what she says.'

Although he'd told me not to worry, I saw the colour drain from his face, and I knew he was thinking exactly the same as me: Could lightning really strike twice?

Sometimes, I forget how much Ash has been through since I was diagnosed. He's so strong, so stoic, such a support – but, while I've been to hell and back, he's been my co-pilot. I'm sure he must be thinking of the worst-case scenario, that he could lose me, 24/7, but he doesn't bother me with his worries. Throughout my lowest points and most gruelling weeks of treatment, I was invariably wrapped up with my own stuff: 'I'm having a bad day, I feel sick, I'm tired, my bones ache, I've got loads to do, I'm being a mum, I need to be mothered myself.'

Looking back, it makes me feel guilty that he was providing me with constant support and yet, during that time, I could offer so very little in return. He's such a strong man, but he's not superhuman. At times, perhaps, I failed to recognize that he was getting a bit worn out by it all too.

Just a week prior to my finding that second lump, I'd caught a rare glimpse of what anguish Ash was actually experiencing. For once, he'd let his real emotions spill out, and it nearly broke my heart.

In theory, after all my excitement about finishing my last chemo session on 22 August, I should have been very upbeat but, after all the build-up to it, I had a distinct sense of anticlimax about the whole thing.

The last dose of chemo was just like every other, which meant I still had to go through days of horrible side effects. I was being sick with horrific regularity, and every bone in my body ached.

When Ash came in from work the day after my final treatment session, Gigi was tucked up in bed, so we both sat on the floor in the lounge and had a cup of tea. Neither of us were talking. I had nothing to say that could make it better. I was tired of pretending that we could go back to being good old Beck and Ash. We weren't that couple any more, and I wasn't the same woman he fell in love with. I felt that my life had disintegrated and, no matter how hard I tried, I couldn't get it back, so what was the point even trying? I didn't know who or what I was, or where he fitted in any more. I could see that Ash was knackered after a long day at work. In the good old, pre-cancer days, Friday nights had had an exciting feel to them. It signalled the start of the weekend – a whole two days for us to spend together as a family. Tonight, it just reminded me of all we had lost.

The radio was on, filling the silence and, as we sat there, the song 'Heaven' came on. It instantly took me back to that moment when Gigi was born. That perfect capsule of time when I'd comforted my newborn daughter after her very first cry and had just been a mother, rather than Rebekah Gibbs, cancer victim. That moment had felt like heaven, and I'd been so optimistic about the future.

Now, six months on, I'd been to hell and back. My relationship with Ash had been tested to the limit, and I wasn't sure there was any more to give. What I found hardest was the fact that I couldn't be the mother I wanted to be. In reality, there would be no more children for me and Ash, no big kitchen table full of childish chatter and tantrums. We couldn't take the risk, and I felt I couldn't even fully enjoy the one chance I had been given.

Listening to the song I'd associated with such happiness and exciting new beginnings overwhelmed me. I started sobbing.

To my surprise, when I looked over at Ash, I saw he was crying too.

It was the first time I'd seen him really cry since April, when I had been told that I definitely had grade-three cancer. Since then, I hadn't seen him break emotionally. I knew he'd had his moments in private, but he was always so together around me.

'Why us, babe?' I asked, through angry, hot tears.

'I don't know,' he said, wiping his eyes. 'I just don't know, Beck. I wish I did.'

You poor bastard, I thought. This is your life too now – living with the fear it could all be over with the discovery of one more lump, dreading every check-up and ache and pain. It's your life sentence too.

As I dialled Rema's number, still touching the lump, I knew Ash was hovering round the corner, listening, waiting to hear.

When I explained what I had found she immediately told me not to panic.

'It's probably scar tissue,' she said. 'I'm seeing you on

Tuesday, so I'll check it out then, but I think it's highly unlikely it's anything to worry about.'

That's what they said last time, I thought to myself, as I put the phone down.

'What did she say, exactly?' Ash asked, and I repeated our short conversation verbatim.

Please don't let there be any more drama, no more operations, treatment, no more cancer, I prayed silently in my head. I don't think I can take any more. As before, we agreed to wait and see before panicking, but that was easier said than done.

On the first Tuesday in September, with my new lump, I headed to Maidstone hospital for my pre-radiotherapy appointment with Rema.

When I arrived, I was taken into a special suite they have for the radiotherapy, and Rema asked me to unbutton my top.

'Let's have a look at this lump then,' she said, getting down to business straight away.

I undressed and sat there anxiously.

'Yep,' she said, feeling the lump thoroughly. 'Scar tissue.'

'Are you sure? I mean, after last time, can I be sure?'

'It would be highly unlikely for a lump that feels like this to turn out to be cancer,' she said.

My mind put at rest, I tried not to move as two nurses and Rema hovered over me taking measurements around where the tumour had been on my left breast and also on my armpit. They have to programme with exact precision where the X-rays are going to attack the tissue. Their primary concern is not to hurt any organs. I was realizing what a natural fidget I am, but I was aware that even the tiniest movement could mean disaster, so I tried to hold my breath and be still.

'We're sure it won't affect your heart,' Rema told me, 'but it could affect one very small corner of your lung. You might get slight scar tissue, but nothing to worry about.'

After all the measurements had been done, there was the novelty of having my very first tattoo done. In fact, I had three – tiny little greeny-blue blobs which pinpointed the exact spot the radiotherapy would hit my skin.

'Can you write "Love" and "Hate" on my knuckles as well?' I joked, trying to lighten the mood. But they were having none of it.

Not long after this appointment, Ash and I decided to take a trip to his parents' holiday home in Marbella. It was a sentimental place that held real memories for us as, the last time we were there, back in March, Gigi had been only seven weeks old, and life had seemed so perfect.

As we stepped into the familiar surroundings of Jen and Rod's villa, I shivered. God, we've been through so much since the last time we were here, I thought, but we're finally getting back on track.

The following day, Jen – or 'Nonny' as she was now better known – had the delight of taking Gigi in the pool for the first time. It was a real spectacle. We all stood round the pool marvelling at Gigi in her little pink swimsuit and rubber ring. I must have taken a million photos. Even though I felt wiped out, I knew it was vital for me to savour all these important moments in her life.

Enjoying all the attention, Gigi grinned goofily, showing off her first tooth, which had appeared a few days before. She was beginning to sit up too. It really made me think about how much time had passed since my diagnosis.

The sun shone every day of our holiday, and it was time for Ash and me to try and claw back some normality, some of the old stardust we used to have.

We had a couple of lunches and a dinner alone so that we could talk about stuff – anything that wasn't to do with medication dosage, radiotherapy side effects, wigs or sickness. Anything other than bloody cancer. As always, his parents really looked after us, and the holiday was the best recuperation I could have wished for. Before we left Spain, I met a friend of Ash's parents called Liz. The previous year, she'd fought breast cancer, and she had written to me when she heard I'd been diagnosed with it, too. We'd exchanged some letters and the odd call and text message, but finally meeting was strange for both of us, and everyone else left the room to give us a chance to catch up.

'I feel like I know you already,' she said, holding my hand.

Well, that set me off – until then, I hadn't cried for weeks! I felt there was a real bond between us. I think you can only really relate to cancer when you've been through it. It's so uncertain, so alien and crushing.

Liz was doing well, and her doctor had told her he expected her to make a full recovery. Hearing that reinforced my sense of optimism that I could beat cancer too.

'I've got a lot to live for, and I'm not going anywhere,' she told me.

I liked her style. 'I'm starting to feel like that again too,' I agreed.

We talked for ages, then we had a big hug and went off to dinner. I was savouring the relaxed rhythm we had here – a world away from endless appointments, examinations and pills.

After her fearless attitude to the swimming pool, I had high hopes for Gigi's first trip to the beach, envisaging big smiles as we dipped her toes in the surf. But, alas, when it came to her *Baywatch* moment, Gigi suddenly became very timid and screamed her head off. I've always preferred the pool myself, too!

By the time we left Marbella after ten glorious days in the sunshine, I'd almost forgotten I had radiotherapy to face once I got back.

When Ash's parents waved us off at the airport, Gigi decided to join in, unleashing a rather floppy hand motion which resembled a relaxed royal wave.

'Look!' I exclaimed to Ash. 'She's waving.'

'Nah,' he replied. 'She's probably got an itchy armpit or something.'

Back in Tunbridge Wells, I felt better than I had in months. Almost four weeks had passed since my last chemo appointment, and every day I was getting more of my energy back. It was like spring creeping in after a long dark winter. You know how every afternoon seems to get a little bit lighter? Well, every day felt like that. My pace seemed to come back, and the depression was lifting.

My first radiotherapy treatment was on 22 September and, driving to Maidstone hospital that morning, I felt peaceful and calm. The forty-five-minute drive gave me plenty of time to think and get 'in the zone'. It felt like I was going for an audition as I psyched myself up for the final stage.

The oncology ward at Maidstone was incredible. It just had this really airy feel about it. Everything was painted a cool blue, and there were plants everywhere. It felt really fresh. Outside, there was this pretty garden area with lovely fountains, tables and chairs, and a coffee bar.

I'd just started flicking through *Hello!* magazine in the waiting room when the nurse called me through a door. Through it was a row of dressing rooms, and I was instructed to pick one and then change into a gown and slippers. When I'd finished getting ready, I was told to leave the room via another door on the other side. I felt like that old cartoon character Mr Benn! (Although I don't recall him ever making an impromptu trip to a radiotherapy unit!) Through that door was a corridor that led me to one of three radiotherapy suites. When I walked in, a nurse turned to me.

'Come in, Rebekah,' she smiled. 'How are we today?'

'Actually, I'm good. Glad to be on the home stretch.'

The room was not dissimilar to an X-ray suite. It had a bed in the middle and bulky metal machinery suspended from the ceiling.

The nurse instructed me to strip to my waist and lie on my back on the bed. Then a radiographer drew lines on my torso and guided me to put one hand on my hip and the other up by my ear.

Next, they lined up the machine above me so that the radiotherapy would target the three sites where the tattoos were, one above my boob under the collarbone, one in the middle of my cleavage and one to the left of my boob, right near where the drain site had been after my lumpectomy.

'Now you need to lie as still as possible,' instructed the radiographer. 'We'll give you three bursts. I'll leave the room for each session, but you'll be able to hear us talking to you through the speaker.'

When they all left the room, I felt very nervous. I knew

that all the careful calculations were to avoid the radiation from damaging my heart, but how could they be 100 per cent sure they would miss it?

Although I couldn't feel a thing, psychologically, I found it all very frightening. I was struggling not to shake, but that first burst of radiotherapy felt like the longest three minutes of my life. I closed my eyes and pictured Gigi laughing. It took away some of the anxiety. I did that in every one of my eighteen sessions.

For three and a half weeks, I had radiotherapy every day from Monday to Friday. The whole process was relentless and, yet again, fighting cancer consumed me. There was the routine of getting everything organized for Gigi every morning to be able to take her to Jen's – packing her bag, making her food and bottles, checking she had everything she might need – and then setting off on the forty-five-minute drive to Maidstone. By the time I'd driven back to Tunbridge, picked up Gigi and settled us in at home, organizing more bottles and food, the day would be practically gone.

I had been desperate to regain control, to get things back to normal, but I had underestimated how exhausting the whole business would be. I knew it delighted Ash to see me coping again but, truth be told, I was knackered. By the second week, things just exploded. It was day nine of my treatment, it was eleven o'clock at night and I was pureeing sweet potatoes, pear and apples and various other nutritious food for Gigi and making up freezer bags. I went into the living room to fetch Gigi's changing bag and found Ash stretched out on the sofa, channel-surfing his way through Sky Plus. Something just went off:

'Ash, do you have any f***ing idea how exhausted I am? Just because I'm not being sick every five minutes, it doesn't mean I'm back to normal. This is hard, Ash, and you aren't helping.'

He looked up at me in amazement. 'What do you mean?' he said. 'I thought you were feeling better? That you wanted to get on with things?'

'Of course I'm feeling better, I couldn't feel worse than I did, but I can't do EVERYTHING!'

He stared at me, stunned by my outburst, and I felt I'd lost any last shred of rationality. The wall of panic and fear was far from down, and now I was taking it out on the person who had been my biggest support. We had slipped back into our old roles too quickly. I still felt broken by the whole experience of battling my way through having cancer, and I wasn't sure we were fighting the same battle any more. It wasn't a given that I would be OK; there was still such a long way to go. Why couldn't he see that?

However, once we (or I!) had cleared the air, something shifted, and we both tried a bit harder to be reasonable for the last leg of the journey. Ticking off the days on the calendar until I finished radiotherapy, I began to feel very satisfied. Cancer is a lonely business; it's an incredibly selfish one too. Looking back, I know I didn't consider Ash's needs enough, but I had to shut something down to be able to get through it.

My radiotherapy continued and, like my days on the chemo ward, before long, there was a real feeling of routine.

I'd always have a natter and a flirt with the car-park attendants, who I'd labelled 'the boys', and I was getting to know a whole new set of nurses, who'd chat to me about Gigi and ask how I was feeling. It was weird but, by this stage, I actually quite enjoyed being able to sit down for fifteen minutes. It was my time to reflect on things.

I know it sounds a bit warped but, during that time when they're drawing on you and measuring everything up, you get gorgeous attention! And, with a small baby, that doesn't happen very often. Also, being at the hospital amongst other cancer patients, there was a real sense of camaraderie.

One day, I walked past a woman wearing a long-haired wig who was being pushed along in a wheelchair. She looked as if she was in pain, but she caught my eye, and we exchanged a knowing look and a smile. I don't know if that woman is going to make it, I thought, but she still had a smile for me.

During the course of my radiotherapy, I was invited to the *Daily Mirror*'s Pride of Britain awards ceremony. This was because I had been doing a weekly column for the newspaper since my diagnosis. Everyone at the *Daily Mirror* has been brilliant throughout, and being invited to the awards was the icing on the cake. I was beside myself with excitement. I'd watched it on TV for years and had always wanted to go. Those stories of courage and bravery regularly reduced me to tears in my living room, so I knew I would have to control myself if I was actually there, especially with all those children and their stories.

I didn't have a clue what I should wear so, in the end, I opted for a classic little black dress, complete with a sparkly skullcap. It was so nice to feel glamorous and have something to dress up for. Ash was staying home to look after Gigi, but he gave me a wolf whistle on my way out – it had been a while since he'd had cause to do that!

The ceremony took place at the London Television Centre, and it was like nothing I'd ever experienced. There were wall-to-wall A-listers like Sir Paul McCartney, Dame Shirley Bassey, Kevin Spacey, and my heroine, Joan Collins. I managed to control my urge to rush over and ask for her autograph, although it was hard!

I was sat on a table with a lovely bunch, including Shirley Bassey's PA, who was adorable.

I knew I had been pretty self-indulgent at times throughout my treatment, so hearing so many stories of selflessness, of surviving through adversity and bravery, really put things into perspective, and I felt incredibly humbled by the winners, from a nine-year-old boy called Nathan, who saved his mum from a knife attack, to my own favourite, Nina Barough, who founded the Walk the Walk charity event. She's raised over £44 million for breast cancer. It's incredible that a normal woman, with just a clear vision and determination has done so much.

Predictably, halfway through the first story, I started crying.

James, my photographer friend, was there, taking pictures for the *Mirror*, and, all of a sudden, he grabbed me. 'Come with me,' he beckoned.

I found myself standing in front of the Prime Minister, Gordon Brown, and his wife, Sarah.

I was really impressed by them. They were so warm and charming, and they both asked me about my experiences of cancer.

'I want to thank you for all the fantastic treatment I've had on the NHS,' I told him. 'The people who've looked after me have been just brilliant.'

The PM looked really chuffed and, inside, I felt secretly smug that I'd made a good impression.

Then James appeared with another familiar face – Trisha Goddard, who had been diagnosed with breast cancer a few weeks after me. As James gathered us all together for a picture, I turned to Gordon and Sarah.

'No kissing!' I joked, referring to the smooch Sarah had given Gordon at the Labour Party conference, which had made headlines the week before.

As I chortled to myself, I noticed no one else was

laughing at my over-familiar banter. Shite. Still, what a fantastic picture for Gigi's memory box!

Afterwards, Trisha and I had a good old chinwag. She was wearing a cute wig and looked incredible. In a mutual love-in, I told her she'd inspired me, because she'd managed to continue her exercise regime and keep up her normal routine, even through her treatment, and she said I'd impressed her by managing with a new baby through it all.

All in all, the emotions of the night definitely took their toll. By 2 a.m., one of my fake eyelashes was starting to droop, and I looked a bit drunk, so I decided to head home.

When I got in at 3 a.m., Ash was sound asleep in bed.

'Ash,' I whispered, selfishly rubbing his arm to wake him. 'I have to tell you about my night!'

Bless him, he sat up and tried his hardest to get excited with me. We had tea and biscuits, while I relayed every bit (including my quip to Gordon and Sarah, to which he replied, 'Jeez, nice one, Beck!'), and then we cuddled up and got two hours' sleep before our darling daughter decided that her early-morning call was happening regardless of whether I'd had a late night or not!

The next morning, as I put on my tracksuit and looked at my black dress and skullcap, discarded from the night before, I was still buzzing. And when I arrived for my radiotherapy session, I could talk of nothing else.

'Have I told you about my old friend Gordon Brown . . .' I joked on the phone to Ash later.

'You're turning into a Pride of Britain bore,' he remarked dryly.

Although I couldn't feel anything happening during the sessions of radiotherapy, as the weeks passed, I noticed I was much tireder than I had been. I had that constantly worn-out feeling, and my chest was beginning to feel sore.

Madeleine had recommended I use aqueous cream, a non-greasy moisturizer that helps to prevent water evaporating from the skin's surface, so I slapped that on every day but, by the second week, my skin was red raw. After every blast it was like I had sunburn.

Even though I knew it would happen, the changes to my body did alarm me, and I had a moment of panic when I noticed that a mole on my left breast had a red shadow on it. Thankfully, it turned out to be no more than a little blister.

As my skin got more and more tender, I tried to be optimistic. 'Good,' I told myself. 'I need this. It means it's working.' But stretching to pick up Gigi made me wince, and the skin across my chest felt really tight, hot and sore.

After fifteen sessions, I switched therapy suites. My last three, intense blasts would concentrate on the lumpectomy area.

By now, I had real war wounds – plenty of blisters, and the radiotherapy had burnt a hole under my armpit. My skin had turned a darker colour, as though I had spent too long in the sun.

On the last day, I breathed a sigh of relief as I dressed for the final time in my little Mr Benn changing room. Stepping outside and walking to the car, I felt tired but very relieved – delighted that it was over and done with and that I'd ticked another box.

That weekend, I left Ash home alone with Gigi and headed off with a friend on a girly weekend to Champneys in the New Forest. I couldn't really swim or use the spa area, because my skin was so sore, but just being there relaxed me. Best of all, I got to watch *Strictly* and the *X Factor* with no distractions, and to sleep for ten glorious hours!

While I was there, I had no word from Ash, and it disturbed me. Was he struggling with the baby but too proud to call? Then, as I watched *Family Fortunes*, the phone rang.

'Babe, she's having a right old whinge,' he said.

So I ran through the checklist: Was she tired? Hungry? Did she have a wet nappy or wind? It eventually transpired that she was one windy baby.

The next morning, Ash called again, this time sounding jubilant. Gigi had just started crawling that week and was into bloody everything!

'I've bought her a play assault course!' Ash announced excitedly.

'Really?' I asked. 'What age is that for then?'

'It says a year old, but I reckon she's a fast learner,' he replied.

'She's only just learned to crawl!' I laughed.

When I got home, it was already packed away in the cupboard. She was lethal on it, and Ash was exhausted from trying to keep up with her.

Later that week, I packed Gigi into the car and drove her down to Devon to see my mum. We had a lovely few days, being ladies who lunch, but when I told Ash I was planning to drive back on the Saturday evening, he stuck his oar in.

'Please don't come back then,' he said. 'I'm not happy about you driving late at night. You know how tired you are after the treatment, and all it takes is one sleepy moment and it's a pile-up, Beck.'

Reluctantly, I agreed to leave Sunday lunchtime instead but, when I hit the M4 near Reading, it all went wrong. We were stuck in slow-moving traffic for ages, with Gigi screaming in protest and the diesel gauge dropping to dangerously near empty. I had to stop at the service station before heading back into the traffic jam once more.

When I finally got home after a seven-hour drive, I was ready to kill Ash. 'I knew I should have left last night,' I yelled at him, once Gigi was tucked in upstairs out of earshot. 'Why do I listen to you? How come you do nothing to help and then interfere when you feel like it?'

It unfolded into a blazing row. In the end, Ash stormed out of the house, and I collapsed on the sofa, exhausted. Blimey, I thought. It's been a long time since we've had a row like that, on equal footing, without him watching his words for the cancer patient. It felt good!

Before Gigi had arrived and I was diagnosed with cancer my rows with Ash were legendary. For some reason, we'd often come to verbal blows in the car while I was driving (I am a very safe but, arguably, slow motorist), and it would always culminate in the same ridiculous sketch being played out:

Ash: 'Let me out of this car!'

Me: 'No, I'm not going to stop the car.'

Ash: 'Let me out, I've had enough. You're a crap driver, Rebekah.'

Well, one evening, all this was going on while we were on the M25.

Oh, you want to get out, do you? I thought, full of rage. I'll show you. I quickly pulled off the motorway, into Clacket Lane services.

'Go on then,' I yelled, screeching to a halt and leaning over him to open the passenger door. 'Bugger off!'

Ash looked at me, a bit stunned, but then, being as stubborn as I am, he spat, 'Fine,' and jumped out, slamming the door behind him.

I drove home. Stormed upstairs, got into bed and fell asleep. I'm not sure how Ash made it the fourteen miles home, but he finally turned up at about 1 a.m. He woke me up, and the row picked up from where we'd left it. We slept in separate bedrooms.

But the next morning, we woke up and we enjoyed a lovely Sunday as if nothing had happened. That was just the nature of our relationship – big bust-ups and then lovely make-ups.

Of course it was the exactly the same scenario after the barney about my nightmare journey back from Devon. Within hours, we were best friends again, and I secretly felt pleased that after Ash tiptoeing around me for months because of the pregnancy, a baby and breast cancer, normal service (and rows) had been resumed in our relationship.

Meanwhile, another twist in the Carry on Cancer epic was looming.

I'd been booked in for a MUGA scan, a non-invasive test which assessed the function of the heart to make sure that the chemotherapy had caused no damage, which involved being given two injections of radioactive dye and then lying on a bed while a moving image was taken of my heart.

I wasn't particularly thrilled that I was going radioactive once more, or that I couldn't have any direct contact with Gigi for two days. I had the injection and, of course, Gigi chose that night not to settle. Ash was on duty, and Gigi was furious that we weren't having our normal bath, bottle, bed routine. She screamed for over an hour as I stood in the bedroom doorway, looking in on Ash, directing him.

'Ash, you've got to hold her really tight and horizontally in your arms like you did when she was small. She'll never go to sleep upright on your shoulder,' I called out. 'Try rocking her harder, she likes that.'

'Rebekah, will you just leave me to it? I have done this before, you know. It's because you're hovering and she knows you're here. She's perfectly fine when we're on our own.'

I retreated and watched him finally get her quiet, rocking her in the nursing chair, and I burst into tears. I imagined being dead, looking down at this bewildered twosome muddling through without me. I imagined wanting to shout down and tell Ash room temp wasn't good enough for her milk, it had to be really warm, that she had to sleep with the light on, that she needed her favourite blanket, not just any old one from the laundry pile. I imagined them getting used to life going on without me. It was heart-breaking.

I pulled myself together, though, and, the following Monday, I was relieved to hear that everything was fine with my heart. I was also given the green light to take part in a new trial of a breast-cancer drug called Lapatinib, which is licensed in the US and will hopefully be in Europe soon as well. Scientists believe it is similar to Herceptin, as it can help reduce the action of an enzyme that causes tumours to grow. It's been decided that I'll take it instead of Herceptin, as part of a worldwide trial. My consultant is hopeful it could be even more effective on me than my previous cocktail of drugs. It's brilliant that there's more hope for sufferers, and things are only going to get better as the research goes on. A few years ago, being diagnosed with cancer would have meant a death sentence for a lot of people, but things are so different now. Charities and the government are putting so much into researching cancer that new treatments and breakthroughs are happening all the time. Hopefully, one day, we'll be at a point where cancer isn't just fought, it's prevented.

However, despite all the good news, the following day, I still woke up in a foul mood. Taking these two new drugs meant another round of tests and hospital appointments in preparation for them but, that day, Ash was busy with work and I had no one else who could babysit. Reluctantly, I took Gigi with me.

She sat in her pushchair as I had the blood tests and then an ECG.

Actually, it was great having her with me. She amused everyone in the waiting room, including me, with her babbles of baby speak and attempts to escape from her pushchair. Despite it being the last place I wanted to take her, there was something comforting about having her with me. She was a real little buddy to me.

Obviously, when I had my chest X-ray, she couldn't come in with me, but the nurses were lining up to look after her. Of course, my little starlet wallowed in the attention and, as soon as I released her from her pushchair, she was showing off shamelessly, manoeuvring herself into a standing position with a big grin, to rounds of applause from the nurses. She was definitely a chip off the old block. Thank goodness, all those results came back clear of any hidden horrors, too, and I was prescribed my drugs. I'm taking six Lapatinib tablets a day, for the next year.

Ten weeks had now passed since the chemo ended, and my hair was well and truly trying to make a comeback. You could no longer see any scalp, and I almost had a pixie crop. Well, almost. If I'm honest about it, I'd gone from being bald to just having a really bad barnet.

'I don't know what you're on about,' Ash insisted. 'It suits you.'

But my fears that he was lying were confirmed when an old college acquaintance spotted me at the train station and eyed my tresses with a look that just said, 'Err, nice haircut.'

Gigi, on the other hand, couldn't give a stuff about my hair – it's my eyelashes she's obsessed with. She eyeballs me with wonder and tries to flick them.

I celebrated my newfound hairiness with a trip to Brighton to see my friend Georgina, whose hair I'd cut off during filming for *Casualty*, in a play called *And Then There Were None*. She was fabulous.

Afterwards, we went for sushi together, looked at cute pics of Gigi and had a good laugh about the to-do I'd made about my broken feng-shui frog all those months before.

'I've had my moments, haven't I?' I admitted.

'Are you feeling more optimistic now?' she asked.

'Yeah, I guess I am,' I said. 'I really feel like the cancer is gone.'

On the drive home, I thought some more about our conversation.

I was feeling good about the future, but also a bit philosophical. There was still a deep, dark place in my mind which contained morbid thoughts about a parallel universe in which the cancer had won and life would go on without me. It made me wonder whether I would see Gigi's first day at school, or her sixteenth, eighteenth or twenty-first birthdays. Would I see my baby's baby? Would I get to be a grandma?

But, whenever I peered inside that world, I'd quickly close the door on it again. I'd never get my head round that prospect, and I just didn't have time to worry about it. Instead, I was going to celebrate the things that needed to be celebrated – and get on and plan my wedding.

After laying on the charm and lots and lots of persuasion, I'd managed to get Ash to set the date for September 2009.

'After seventeen years, he's finally going to make an honest woman of me,' I'd whooped down the phone to Michelle. 'It's going to be a pink extravaganza. Jordan and Peter have nothing on me!'

Primarily, I wanted to celebrate with all my friends and

family. I had no idea when I'd next get all those people I loved in the same room again, so it was really any excuse for a party.

I guess my next big celebration will be when I'm forty, in five years' time. It's scary, and I don't want to wish those five years away, but I hope it coincides with the time I get the all clear. You need these markers to guide the way, things to hold on to. Whenever Ash and I talk about the future, it's only ever positive. And, with our little girl causing mayhem wherever she goes, it certainly keeps us upbeat and rushed off our feet.

For Gigi's first Christmas, we flew to Marbella and spent it with Ash's parents.

I cannot tell you how exciting it was to put together her first ever stocking from Santa. She loved it. Admittedly, it was the wrapping paper rather than the gifts inside that excited her but, still, to see her grinning with delight and wrecking the tree was magical.

My hair was still growing back, and it was a relief to get to the stage where, to look at me, no one would know I'd been ill at all.

We spent New Year's Eve at this amazing hotel, tucking into seven courses, with a group of ten of our family and friends. Jen, always the angel, insisted on sloping off early with Gigi, so Ash and I could carry on celebrating. Just before midnight, I gazed around at everyone. They were all looking so happy and excited about the future.

'We got there, babe,' Ash said, cuddling me. 'We did it, sweetheart!'

I would have shed a tear if I hadn't been so concerned with trying to shove twelve grapes down my neck, one with each chime of the clock at midnight. It was a Spanish tradition, and was supposed to bring good luck.

After I'd nearly choked, I grinned at Ash. 'Roll on 2009,' I mumbled, trying to stop the juice dribbling down my chin.

When Gigi hit her first birthday, I knew I had so much to celebrate. Every day, she becomes more and more of a character. She really is my everything, the centre of my world and, with every breath I have in me, she'll always be the most important thing on my mind.

Although I am being positive, I have prepared for her life with or without me. If the worst happens, I know what schools I want her to go to, I know the way I want her brought up, and I will ensure that she is completely showered with love.

I am encouraging Ash more and more to share in her little routines – he knows her favourite bedtime songs and picture books, knows she doesn't like spinach and will only have milk out of her special bottle. If I'm not here, Ash knows where I'm coming from. He knows my ethics and the values I want instilled in my little girl. Thankfully, we share the same outlook on all the important stuff.

I want her to have hobbies – I had my dancing, and Ash

had boxing, so neither of us was ever bored. We were both encouraged to believe we could do it. Ash was a good boxer, and it was strong grounding for him. He didn't smoke or drink like other boys in his group because he was focusing on his training every night. I had that dedication and focus, too, with my dancing, and that's what we want for our baby: goals, dreams and fun.

My cancer threw a spanner in the works, it slowed us down and tried to stop us. And, the fact is, we still have a lot of unknown territory to charter. I'll take my tablets for twelve months, I'll be examined every year for five years. I may get the news I'm in remission, the cancer may come back – but I'll always dread the check-ups and mammograms and worry about every little ache and pain.

But we still have all our dreams. They haven't been shattered. I did want more children, but I won't have them now, I can't risk it. So we'll look into fostering and adoption and, who knows, we may get our kitchen table full of children, like I'd hoped.

The funny thing is, even before cancer came into our lives, I'd thought about fostering. I was inspired by Ash's mum, who'd spent a lot of years growing up in a children's home.

She's got these fantastic fond memories of a couple who came and took her and her sister home to their house for Christmas. They lived by the seaside, and she says that holiday stayed with her for years, gave her faith that she could have a life of her own, make it what she wanted. I think that is so special. That's why I always try and remember how important it is that we do have our dreams. They don't have to be wild and wonderful, but they do give us something to work towards. Together, we talk about holidays, moving, being financially secure, Gigi's education – anything but the worst-case scenario.

I've got my own dreams, too.

There are shows I still want to do, things on my career wishlist I want to achieve, although it isn't my top priority any more. Before, my work dominated everything. I compromised things I wouldn't have if I'd known what was coming, but hindsight is a wonderful thing.

We have to assume all will be good, until we hear otherwise, and I pray that day never comes. But I have realized I can't live in fear; it would be a waste of the second chance I have been given. I can't live the rest of my life fearing death.

I'll do all I possibly can to stay healthy and stave the cancer off but, if I'm not here for much longer, I know I picked the best man I could to be my daughter's father.

If I'm honest with myself, at times, I've doubted me and him. There have been moments where I was desperate for commitment and he didn't deliver, or when I've wondered if our relationship is as good as it could be, but I have always known that I have been loved.

Ash will give Gigi everything. He has got that love, that

warmth, that discipline. She won't be spoilt, but he'll give her the future, he'll give her the dreams, he'll tell her to go for it, just as I would. Being an actress can be tough. It's not all green rooms and hair and make-up – you do get a lot of knocks, and you don't always get the gig. But Ash is always bolstering me, and I know I'm lucky – he has always looked after me. He has always told me: 'Beck, don't care, just get in there and do it. You don't need the job, I'll look after you for the rest of your life. You do it because you love it.' I just love him for that, because he's given me such freedom to make choices and hold out for the good jobs.

I want Gigi to have that fighting spirit that I think Ash and I share. Things haven't always come easy for us, and I'm proud that that makes us the people we are today.

I want her to find out what makes her tick, what excites her, where her talent lies. And I'd like her to get married and have children, because I think it's just the best thing I've ever done. I do often wonder why I waited until I was thirty-five. She's bloody amazing! But, as Ash and I always say, if we'd done this ten years ago, it wouldn't have been the same, and it wouldn't have been Gigi. It had to be now.

If the worst comes, and the cancer stalks me to the end, I won't dwell on the things I'll miss, I'll try and focus on what I can still enjoy, how much happiness and fun I can cram into my remaining time with Gigi.

And I know if Ash goes and finds another woman, he'll pick a good one. I know he'll find someone to look after him and Gigi, someone who'll love her as much as he does. And that is fine by me, because I wouldn't want him to be lonely.

If I can't be there, then all I want for them is to be happy.

I always remember something Jen said to me when Gigi was born. 'You only borrow these children,' she said. 'They're not yours to keep.' So, all I can do is my best for Gigi and leave her to make her own way in the world.

I want to be by her side and help her through all those special occasions – her first day at school, her first period, her first boyfriend, her first job, her first baby – but if, God forbid, I'm not, I will write those letters to help her. I will do everything I can to prepare her.

I will tell her about being strong, about getting back up when she falls, not taking no for an answer and about banging on those doors. I'll tell her to be happy.

'If you want something, go for it,' I'll say. 'Because life is short and precious and you have to make the most of every day.'

To my darling girl,

There is so much I want to say to you, so I am writing this letter just in case I'm not here to tell you myself.

I am looking at you right now – you're fast asleep,

and I'm about to give you your favourite dream feed. I can't believe that as I give you your bottle you sleep through the whole thing! But you do and you look so peaceful.

You're like clockwork – sleeping through until 5 a.m., when you wake and I lift you out of your cot and into bed with me for a cuddle. It's our special routine, we lie there until 7 a.m. dozing, and then we get up for breakfast. Of course I've broken every rule in the book by doing this but, since I was diagnosed, I've ditched the baby guides. We do things our way now. I don't know who gets more comfort out of it, me or you.

Did you know that, when you sleep, you clench your thumbs in your hands just like Daddy does?

You and Daddy are very similar, and not just in looks. I'm sure as you get older you'll have your moments with each other, but love him. Look after him, take time for him, be patient and cuddle him – just like he does for you.

I picked you a great daddy. He is an enigma. He's kind, strong, intelligent, and he's my best friend. And he will be yours if you want him to be.

Learn from your daddy, Gigi, he has your best interests at heart. And when you pick a partner, think of all the qualities that you most admire and make sure he has them.

You are blessed to have such wonderful grand-parents and godparents. They are there to love and guide you. Turn to them and trust them, but also trust yourself.

Dare to dream, sweetheart, as without dreams we are nothing. I have fulfilled lots of mine, and having you was my biggest one of all.

Motherhood is the best role I have ever had and, when the time is right for you, embrace it if you can. Remember, it's all about love. You are full of love, my little Pookie No No – I have no idea where that came from, but it's your special nickname! You always look up expectantly when I call you it, laughing at your silly mummy.

You are a kind soul, Gigi. It sounds strange, but it hasn't just been me caring for you since you were born. Sometimes you look at me when I am crying with such tenderness and understanding, it breaks my heart. But I want you to know how much strength you have given me, through the toughest of times. I'll never forget how you stroked my head on the day that I started to lose my hair from the chemotherapy. It was like you just knew.

Throughout your very first summer, I was exhausted from my treatment and, most afternoons, you came to bed with me to keep me company, and we cuddled up all cosy and safe.

I love that we can comfort each other. When you snuggle up with me in bed in those early mornings, you hold my hand tightly and then you drift back to sleep, both of us feeling safe and secure.

You are everything I could wish for in a daughter, Gigi, and if I am only going to have one baby, I am so glad it is you. I am proud to be your mummy. You laugh when I laugh, you yawn when I yawn and you dance when I dance. Like me, you love people. A stranger told me the other day how outgoing and sociable you are for such a young baby. It made me realize that, sometimes, I forget to really look at you when I'm feeling ill or down or scared about what the future holds. But when I do look at you, my love, I discover a new gift from you each time.

You are one of life's angels, Gigi. Be the best you can be. No one else's idea of best – just yours. That will be enough.

Don't forget to smell the roses, sweetheart. I'll be with you.

With all my love and hugs for ever,

Mummy xxx

Acknowledgements

There are so many people who've offered me amazing support throughout my battle against breast cancer.

Firstly, thank you to all my friends for helping me through my journey, especially Mich and James, who encouraged me to share this story.

Thank you to my family for your love and support. Mum, Dad, Alan and Jen, you have all been amazing. Thank you for the constant care you've given the three of us. Jen, thank you so much for having Gigi at the drop of a hat and, for all your financial support – we really couldn't have done it without you. Mum, thank you for looking after me and for the amazing home cooking.

Victoria, my neighbour, you've been so kind and like a second mum to me. I really appreciate all you've done.

Thank you to Simon, Amber and George for your positive attitude from the very beginning – it was invaluable.

Thank you to Cancer Research UK for giving me inspiration, and to all the staff at Maidstone and Tunbridge Wells NHS Trust and Spire Hospital in Tunbridge Wells. I'd also like to thank Cancer Care for helping to support me and the book. I'd like to thank Mr Tim Williams, Dr Rema Jyothirmayi and all the nurses who cared for me on the oncology ward and during my chemo and radiotherapy – particularly Jo, Lou, my Macmillan nurse Maggie and Anne Phillips my trial nurse.

Many thanks to my friend and acupuncturist Dr B and also to everyone of the *Daily Mirror* for all your support.

At Headline, my publishers, I would like to thank my brilliant editor, Carly Cook, for her humour and energy, but most of all her total belief that this story would make a book. And to Josh Ireland, Emily Furniss, Sarah Day and Jo Liddiard for all their hard work. I'd also like to thank Charlotte Ward, who's been my mentor and wordsmith and has listened as I've laughed or cried since day one of this journey.

Most of all Ashley, my soulmate, thank you for always being there and, last but not least, my little girl, Gigi. Thank you, sweetheart, for giving me something to live for.